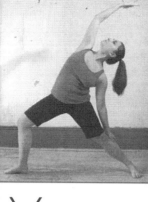

# Yoga

# For
# Singers

Freeing Your
Voice and
Spirit Through
Yoga

**Linda Lister**

# Yoga For Singers

## *Freeing Your Voice and Spirit Through Yoga*

**BY LINDA LISTER**

Photography by Maryann Bates

Cover Design by Dave Harper

Interior Design by Dave Harper and Rommel Alama

©2011 by Linda Lister. All rights reserved.

ISBN #: 978-1-257-09212-3

*To singers everywhere:*
*may you find solace*
*in your song*
*and in yourself.*

TABLE OF CONTENTS

# Table of Contents

# Preface

Once relegated to new age stores and hippie culture, yoga has
become a familiar part of mainstream American culture. Yoga mats
can be found for sale at mass-market stores like Walmart, and
numerous books on yoga line the shelves at Barnes & Noble and
Borders. Still, I thought my opera workshop class might be somewhat resistant when I began to incorporate some yoga poses into
our physical warm-up. To my surprise and delight, the students
took great enjoyment in the challenges and rewards of yoga. When
they asked that I teach a class on the subject, I began to think about
how yoga was of particular interest and relevance to singers. These
thoughts guided my development of the class and are the origin of
this book. I am grateful to the vocal coaches, voice teachers, and
editors who read early drafts and graciously gave feedback and
input on this book. A special thank you goes to photographer Maryann Bates for capturing the antics of my yoga models (the affable
Tré Appleby, flexible Megs Free, genial Jasmine Habersham, and
the marvelous Megan Cone) and bringing our yoga practice to life
in an artful way.

Linda Lister, D.M.A.

# Introduction

*ANXIETY n. An abnormal and overwhelming sense of apprehension and fear often marked by physiological signs (as sweating, tension, and increased pulse), by doubt concerning the reality and nature of the threat, and by self-doubt about one's capacity to cope with it.\**

*FREE adj. Not determined by anything beyond its own nature. Not obstructed, restricted, or impeded. Determined by the choice of the actor or performer.\**

---

\* These definitions are from (www.merriamwebster.com).

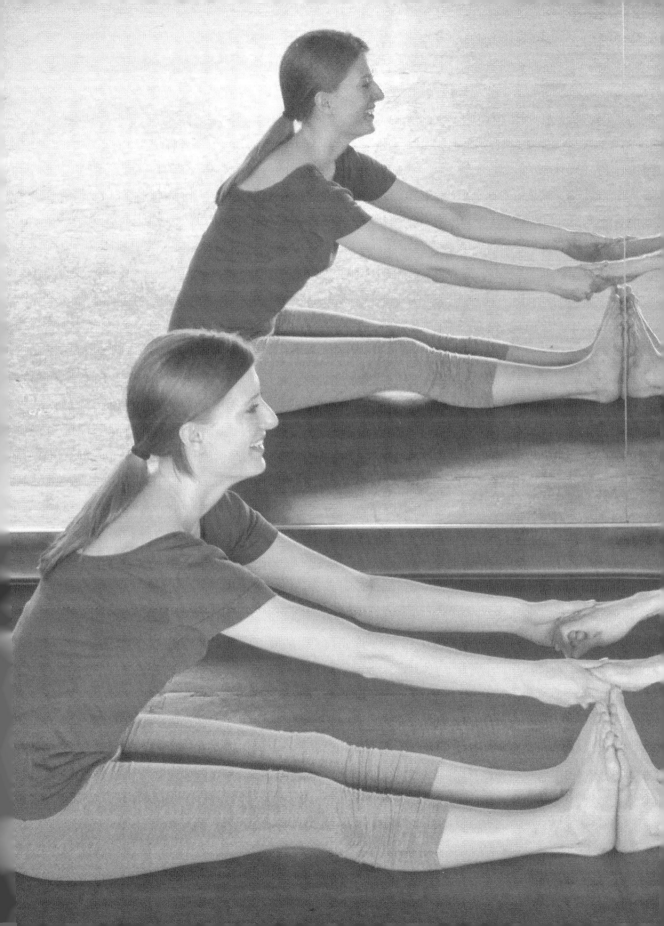

*"Singers should practice yoga. It teaches you great concentration. When you sing on the great stages of all the great theaters of the world, including those giant halls on the Met tour up to ten thousand in capacity, you have to have nerves of steel."*

—**Mario Sereni**, *baritone*

Before I was a singer I was dancer. Studying at the Ballet West Academy, I discovered the beauty and rigor of ballet. During the class warm-up done at the ballet barre, exacting positions are attempted and repeated in order to train the body to perform the exquisite yet in some ways unnatural art of ballet. Despite having considerable flexibility and extension, I was never able to achieve the perfect positions due to less than ideal hip turnout and foot arches (like the character Jody Sawyer in the film *Center Stage*). Although I continued to dance in musical theatre productions and in my college dance company, once I entered graduate school at the Eastman School of Music, I abandoned my dancing dreams to focus on singing.

But I missed the joy and freedom of movement. Once I started teaching voice at the collegiate level, I dabbled in hobbies and classes, trying to find an outlet for my need for movement. After taking swing dance, tai chi, kickboxing, and Pilates, I finally took a yoga class. Suddenly I felt at home. Yoga provided physical, emotional, and even spiritual release for me. My teacher guided me through the specifics of asanas or poses. I quickly learned that – in a thrilling contrast to my experiences with ballet – yoga demands no "perfect position" and my body was not criticized for failing to achieve an elusive standard of perfection. I found that yoga is not about how you look in the poses but how you feel after doing them. Instead of my body serving the poses, the poses served and fed my body. This breakthrough brought with it a great feeling of personal liberation and peace, which not only improved the quality of my life, but was helpful in my other pursuits, particularly my singing.

Like many singers and performers, I still suffer from moments of stage fright. A singer's ability to sing well is wholly dependent on his/her ability to breathe well, and performance anxiety usually involves an elevated heart rate leading to shallow breathing. I found myself backstage before performances doing breathing exercises from yoga class in an attempt to combat my body's flight response. While those around me may have found it odd to see an opera singer in a formal dress with her hands on the floor in Downward-Facing Dog, I had found a tool to help alleviate the stress of singing in front of a large audience.

Thus it is my goal to share with other singers the tools that yoga can provide to help improve their physical and emotional well-being, to assist in their alignment and breathing, to bring both freedom and control to their singing, and to manage the anxiety of performing with the most personal of instruments – their voices.

*"Yoga is a metaphor for life. You find yourself in very humiliating situations, but you can't judge yourself. You just have to breathe, and let go. It is a workout for your mind, your body and your soul."*

*—Madonna*

# Author's Note:

Before beginning any new exercise program, check with your physician. Also, beginners are best advised to start their yoga practice with a capable instructor. (See the glossary for information on finding a teacher via an online directory of accredited instructors.)

Some singers, especially those with musical theatre backgrounds involving dance and movement, will be more comfortable with yoga practice at first, but all singers need to cultivate body awareness and can benefit from the kinesthetic learning, stress relief, and breathing techniques yoga provides.

# DON'T GET A SORE THROAT FROM YOUR YOGA MAT!

Sore muscles are okay after yoga class, but you don't want to end up with a sore throat from your yoga mat. Most gyms and health clubs provide communal yoga mats and blocks for students to use in class. While this may seem like a useful convenience and money saver, you may spend a lot more in medicine if you catch something from using the handy public mat. Without proper cleaning, communal mats can harbor bacteria and/or viruses. To be safe, check with your gym on their procedure for cleaning and disinfecting mats. But the best option is to bring you own mat. (Especially for Bikram or sweaty yoga!) Of course, you should also take care to clean your mat. Hand wash and air dry with a mild detergent every few weeks or so. After each use, use a mat-cleaning spray to keep it fresh-smelling. (You can make your own by mixing three drops of tea tree oil, two drops of peppermint oil, and two drops of lavender oil in distilled water.)

Basic yoga mats can range in price from $10-20 at sporting goods and discount stores (i.e. Tar-get) and can even be found at drugstores (Walgreens, GNC). Most mats are 24" wide and 68" long. Standard depth is 1/8" but you can pay more for a thicker mat if you prefer. Eco mats are also becoming popular, since they are in line with the yogic philosophy of natural, sustainable living. Made from biodegradable, renewable rubber and free from latex, PVC, chloride and glue, eco mats are usually $50-70. Blue and purple seem to be the most common colors for yoga mats but you can find one in a color that fits your personality and practice. I am a fan of Gaiam's premium mats: their elegant prints in soothing colors provide an aesthetically pleasing environment for my yoga practice (and give me another outlet for artistic expression!).

A neat new development is a Gaiam yoga mat which has a built-in audio speaker. Simply hook up your iPod or MP3 player to the mat and you can practice or lead a class without a separate sound system.

# 1

## Hatha Yoga: Iyengar Alignment and Kundalini Energy

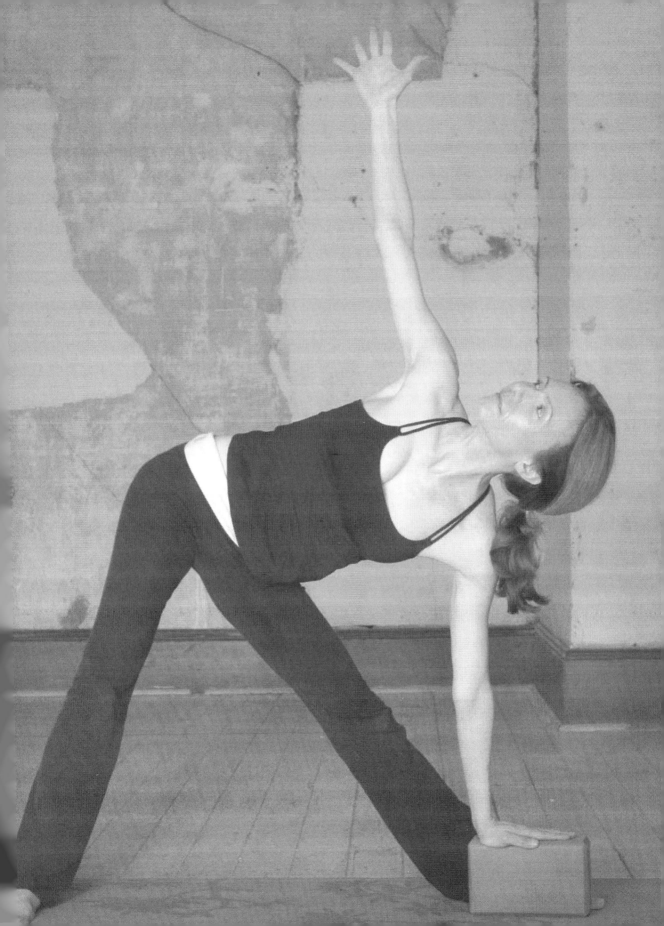

*"A lot of my yoga practice has to do with silencing that voice that would have you come out of the posture or not remember the words or think negative thoughts or dwell on things that aren't important. It kind of speaks to the psychology of singing."*

—**Measha Brueggergosman**, *soprano and certified Bikram Yoga Teacher, Classical Singer magazine, March 2011*

*YOGA* n. (Sanskrit) union

The practice of yoga began over five thousand years ago. Originating in the Hindu Vedic tradition, it was first used as a means of uniting the individual's body, mind and soul, thus uniting them with the Divine. There are six main branches of yoga, but some are of less relevance to singers. For instance Jnana yoga focuses on the path to spiritual wisdom, while Karma or service yoga deals with individual actions and their outcome. Tantra yoga has gained some notoriety as of late thanks to a fascination with its sensual properties, but it will not be part of this discussion. Neither will Bhakti or devotion yoga with its prayerful focus on the Divine. Instead, the emphasis will be on **Hatha yoga**, or physical yoga. The Sanskrit word *hatha* is the union of two other words, *ha* (sun) and *tha* (moon). Thus, hatha yoga implies the union of seemingly opposite forces to create balance and harmony. Singers must also strive for a similar balance: the union of artistry and music with technique and the physical body. The union of these syllables creates a word literally meaning "forceful." Of course no singers should be forcing or straining as part of their performance or as part of their yoga practice. Instead, the principles of Hatha yoga embody physical vigor and power as elements that can enhance and embolden healthy, dynamic singing. [For more information, see the glossary on styles/school of yoga.]

Hatha yoga has many branches as well. Some systems of hatha yoga are not as helpful for singers. The extreme rigor of Ashtanga or power yoga and the increasingly popular Bikram or Hot yoga are not as friendly to singers, who are not usually dancers or athletes and who value hydration as part of maintaining the health of their voices. However both the Iyengar and Kundalini branches are of particular interest to singers, thus this book will focus on a blend of these two schools.

## BROADWAY DIVAS ON BIKRAM YOGA: HOT OR TOO HOT?

"I went to a lot of Bikram Yoga so I could be ready to wear some shells on stage."
–Soprano **Sierra Boggess** on getting cast as
*The Little Mermaid* on Broadway

"Bikram yoga helps keep the weight down. Yoga's a very spiritual thing to do anyway."
–**Audra McDonald**, Tony Award-winner for *Ragtime*, *Carousel* and *Master Class*

"Idina [Menzel] was really into Bikram yoga, which is very, very hot. She did it every day. I tried it, and it kind of made me want to throw up. It's so hot!"
–**Julia Murney**, Elphaba in the national tour of *Wicked*

For more about hatha yoga, read the practice's classic 15th century manual, the Hatha Yoga Pradipika. http://www.yogavidya.com/Yoga/HathaYogaPradipika.pdf

# Iyengar: Alignment

The Iyengar style of yoga comes from the teachings of guru Bellur Krishnamachar Sundararaja (BKS) Iyengar (b. 1918). Iyengar's focus is on the eight aspects of the Yoga Sutras of Patanjali, an ancient yoga philosopher or school of thought. (Scholars are still debating whether Patanjali was a single author or compiler, and whether the Sutras date from 2nd century BC or 5th century AD.) The four aphorisms of this group which are most helpful to singers are:

• Asanas: body postures/poses
• Pranayama: breath control
• Dharana: focus/concentration
• Dhyana: meditation

What makes Iyengar yoga unique is its emphasis on alignment of the body in postures (asanas), the use of props to help achieve ideal alignment, and the sequencing of the asanas. Proper body alignment is of supreme importance to singers. Without proper alignment, the breathing mechanism can be compromised, and poor posture can also cause the singer to look slouched and insecure. The use of yoga blocks and/or straps achieves ideal form in students of varying degrees of experience and flexibility. Iyengar seems to have a particular affinity for musicians and he alludes to them a number of times in his writings. In *Light on Yoga*, perhaps the definitive yoga book of the 20th century, he likens yoga's union of body and mind to "a great musician becoming one with his instrument and the music that comes from it."[1] It is not surprising then, that the Iyengar style has such utility for singers. His insights into the exigencies of the artistic personality are quite telling indeed.

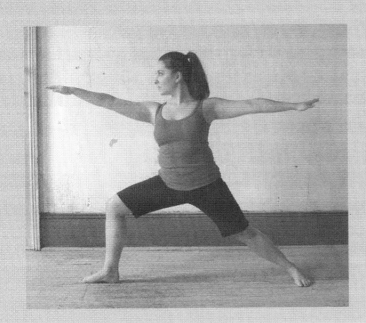

Incorporating yoga into my vocal training has been immensely helpful to my growth as a singer and performer. To me, yoga is about connecting the mind, body, and breath so that everything works together as one, and that connection is also what creates a good performance. I've learned to trust that my body will know what to do and how to do it, which allows me to get out of my own way and focus on the emotion and story of a song, rather than nerves.

-*Megan Cone, ensemble, national tour of "All Shook Up"*

*Many actors, acrobats, athletes, dancers, musicians and sports-men also possess superb physiques and have great control over the body but they lack control over the mind, the intellect and the self. Hence they are in disharmony with themselves and one rarely comes across a balanced personality among them.*[2]

So it is that Iyengar's method develops and encourages optimal alignment not only of the body but also of the mind. His sequence of asanas is uniquely positioned to tone and tune the singer's physical instrument while also training and attuning the singer's mental capabilities to achieve mental clarity and harmony. With the ability to maintain a confident and calm psyche, the singer is then able to present a more focused and revelatory performance onstage as well as a more content and correspondingly more balanced presence off-stage.

# YOGA AND SPIRITUALITY

The origins and influences of yoga are allied with both Hinduism and Buddhism, even Sufism. Initially, some of my opera students were scared that practicing yoga would be sacrilegious to their Christian beliefs, or that physicality should not be part of spirituality. Modern hatha yoga is physical yoga. It is taught in gyms, spas, and yoga studios not churches and is not meant to be a religious experience. Instead it is meant for exercise, stress relaxation and relaxation.

I have not included a sacred component in my yoga teaching, but I have told students that they are welcome to bring their own spirituality to meditation if they so choose. Like prayer, meditation involves focusing one's attention to a different level of awareness. But unlike prayer, meditation need not involve faith or worship, but it could if one chooses.

In fact, there is a growing movement which explores Christ-centered yoga practice. Proponents include Yahweh Yoga (www.yahwehyoga.org) which cites this Bible verse from Corinthians: "Do you not know that you yourselves are God's temple and that God's Spirit lives in you? For God's temple is sacred, and you are that temple." They seem to recognize that taking care of the body is not an irreverent, purely sensual thing but something necessary for good health and wellness.

## Kundalini: Energy

A tall, energized spine is essential in establishing ideal alignment for good singing. Kundalini yoga centers on the idea of harnessing the energy of the spine. Represented by *shakti* or a serpent, this nerve energy is thought to lie in the lower end of the spine like a snake. This coiled or *kundalini* energy is both physical and psychic and thus affects both the body and the spirit. It is not hard to imagine that the central nervous system housed in the spinal column could be a great source of energy. If you view your spine as an extension of your nervous system stemming from your unique brain, then it is also not so difficult to imagine your spine as your own unique instrument. Kundalini energy is viewed as "our latent spiritual potential"[3] and the practice of Kundalini yoga attempts the journey of raising kundalini or awakening and actualizing your true potential, your full consciousness, and deepest enlightenment. So your mother was really onto something when she told you to stand up straight!

For many centuries a highly secretive and guarded tradition, the practice of Kundalini yoga was brought to the west in 1969 by Yogi Bhajan (né Harbhajan Singh Puri, 1929-2004). Kundalini energy is thought to be awakened and activated through energy centers or meridians called chakras (wheels). The intricacies of chakra study have provided the subject for many previous books and will not be the main focus of this study. Indeed the complexities of Kundalini yoga may seem at first somewhat daunting; however the practice's coordination of breath and movement is a natural connection to breathing for singers. Furthermore, Kundalini's mixture of breathing, chanting, mantras, and mudras makes it a wonderful means of combining singing and meditation. In addition, the importance of a free-flowing, uncoiled spine is central not only to good health but to the proper alignment for good vocal technique.

*"Yoga makes me feel like I can do anything."*
— **Lady Gaga**

Yoga is about breathing through physical challenges, and it can help singers learn to breathe to control their nerves in the physical and emotional challenges of live performance.

# 2

# Pranayama:
# Breath and
# Life Control

*"When the breath is steady or unsteady,*
*so is the mind, and with it the yogi."*

— Hatha Yoga Pradipika

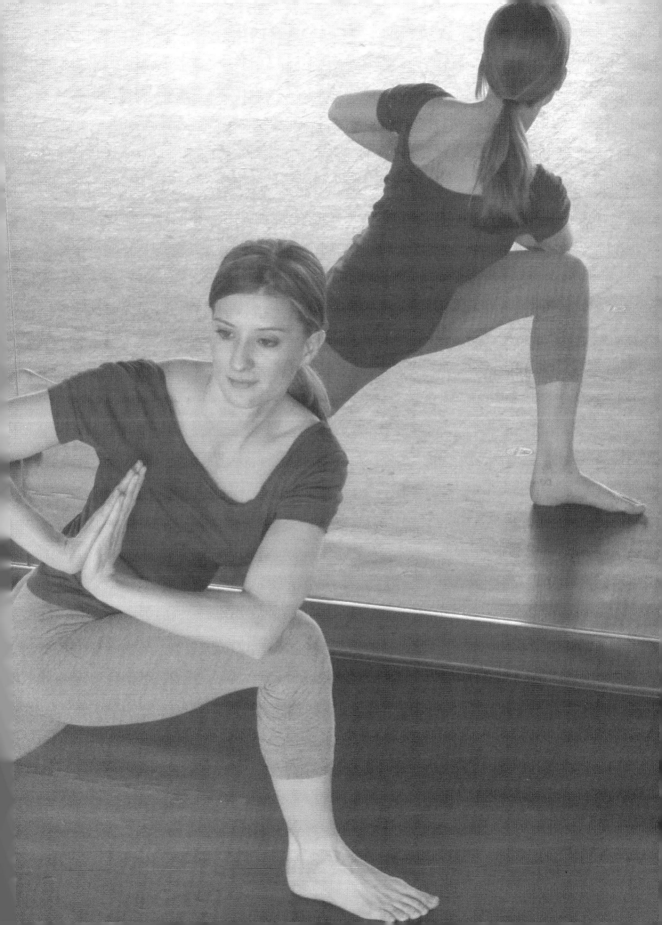

Pranayama means "life control" or "breath control," an interesting double meaning. A singer's ability to sing well is wholly dependent on the singer's ability to breathe well. A classical singer is often required to deliver musical phrases of very long, sometimes even Herculean duration. (Some key phrases from Brahms's "Die Mainacht" and the Strauss "Four Last Songs" come to mind.) And singers in the realms of musical theatre and pop music must frequently sing while performing intricate, highly aerobic choreography. Just imagine the cast of the Broadway musical *A Chorus Line* singing "One" while doing repeated high kicks, or think of the cardiovascular demands on Beyoncé ( a reported yoga practitioner) performing songs like "Single Ladies" or "Crazy in Love" in concert. It is not surprising then, that even with more advanced students, voice teachers continue to emphasize the importance of good breath management. Learning the proper coordination and developing the strength and freedom to maintain optimal breathing for singing is one matter, and then there is the irksome, troubling, and sometimes debilitating, negative impact that stage fright can have on breath control.

Even with substantial training and skill, many singers still suffer from performance anxiety. In what is a normal and scientifically documented occurrence, the excitement, nervousness and perceived risk of public performance can all trigger the fight or flight response.[a] This stress response is manifested in familiar physical reactions such as accelerated heart rate, high/shallow breathing, and dry mouth, all very detrimental conditions for any singer. It can cause even a talented, well-trained singer to "choke" or fold under pressure. Therefore, the successful singer must not only master good breath management but must also learn to combat the biology of the stress response in order to achieve good breath management in high pressure performance situations.

a For more scientific background on the fight or flight response, visit the website of physician Neil F. Neimark: (www.thebodysoulconnection.com/EducationCenter/fight.html). Some interesting books on the topic include: *A Clinical Guide to the Treatment of the Human Stress Response* by George S. Everly and Jeffrey M. Lating, and *Neural Path Therapy: How to Change Your Brain's Response to Anger, Fear, Pain, and Desire* by Matthew McKay and David Harp.

## YOGA ON TOUR:

While on tour, jazz singer **Diana Krall** requests a separate backstage yoga room.

Soprano **Nicole Cabell** packs yoga DVDs when she departs for an out-of-town opera gig.

During the five-year run of her Las Vegas show at Caesars Palace, **Celine Dion** had a personal yoga/meditation instructor and Thai Yoga Massage therapist.

"Doing yoga on the road was really a life-saver, and a life-changer. It helped me to approach my day differently. It kept me focused and gave me more control over the way I divided my energy."
–singer/songwriter **Sheryl Crow**, Yoga Journal September 2000

Although there are certainly a number of schools of thought on the subject and a multitude of pedagogical approaches, breathing for singing involves what is most commonly known as breath support. A form of very conscious respiration, breath support involves using the rib and abdominal muscles to lean out or support to extend exhalation. Singing is essentially controlled exhalation while one phonates or makes vocal sound. During inhalation, the goal is expansion in the lower abdomen as the lungs expand downward, filling with air as the diaphragm also descends and pushes some digestive organs forward. This is why many singers find it uncomfortable to sing on a full stomach. No singer wants to be burping in the middle of a flashy cadenza or during a climactic high note! (Unless he is playing the title role in *Shrek: the Musical...*) As vocal pedagogue James McKinney ably states, "perhaps the best way to gain control of the exhalation is to try to maintain the expansion around the middle of the body"[4] as one begins and

*"Every time I take a [yoga] class, I want to cry. I don't know if it's because I'm relaxing, or if it's that by the end of the class, your body can do things it couldn't do in the beginning, so you feel accomplished and emotional. It's therapeutic."*

—*Beyoncé Knowles*,
*sixteen-time Grammy Award-winning R & B singer*

continues to sing. The idea is to resist against the diaphragm instead of assist in expelling the air from the lungs. However this resistance needs to be properly actualized so as not to create stiffness or unwanted tension in the body. I am fond of the Italian term for support, *appoggio* (from the verb *appoggiare* meaning "to lean"), because it implies a dynamic and elastic muscular action and avoids negative words such as "push," "press," and "lock," all terms I consciously avoid in my voice teaching. These words imply rigidity in the body which can hinder breath flow and create deleterious tension. Pranayama, or yoga breathing, emphasizes that breath energy should always be flowing through the body since breath is life. This concept of fluidity is so helpful in eliminating body tension and encouraging continuity and consistency in the breath cycle. Continuity and consistency of breath lead to greater breath control, an imperative for any successful singer. And yoga breathing techniques can help provide a solid grounding for improving breath control for singers.

Good alignment is essential to good breathing. Before listing the qualities of efficient breath management, let's first review the important postural details necessary to achieve it. These need to be established before and maintained during the entirety of the breath cycle:

• A long back of the neck on which the head freely rests

• A high sternum and open upper chest

• A broad shoulder yoke in which the shoulders are rolling back and are not elevated

• A wide, expansive rib cage in which the intercostals are engaged

• A long, energized spine with awareness of all the vertebrae

• The stacking of hips, knees, and ankles in line with the spinal column

Common incorrect tendencies will include bringing the head forward off the neck, pressing down on the sternum, bringing the shoulders up, collapsing the ribs, and/or curving the spine, especially near the ends of challenging phrases. After checking on alignment, then you can begin to think about the key elements of good breathing habits for singing:

- A low, slow, and silent inhalation
- A low abdominal expansion as the lungs expand and the diaphragm descends
- An exhalation involving muscular resistance of the abs and intercostals
- A recovery which begins the next inhalation and continues the breath cycle

In Iyengar's method, the asanas are used not only as means of establishing good alignment but are also useful in building good breathing habits: "the lungs, the diaphragm and the intercostal muscles must be trained and disciplined by asanas so that the breath moves rhythmically"[5] thereby coordinating and establishing the breath cycle. You should think of maintaining the cycle of inhalation (puraka) and exhalation (rechaka) as you hold a single asana or as you move through vinyasas. Remember that prana is not only breath but life! Whether moving in a complicated power yoga vinyasa or standing calmly in Mountain pose, the goal is to keep breath energy – and thus <u>life</u> energy – flowing vitally through the body before you begin to sing.

*"What's wonderful about yoga is there's not a sense of achievement, it's more a sense of acceptance…this incredible feeling of tranquillity. The accomplishment is relaxation rather than drive."*

— ***Frederica von Stade**,*
*mezzo-soprano,*
*LA Times interview, 1990*

# PRANA FOR PERFORMANCE

I've been singing since I was three, and ever since then it's been hard to get me to shut up. Singing is an incredibly important part of my life – it's my form of expression, my chosen art form, what keeps all the emotions inside of me from bubbling over and exploding. I came to college knowing I wanted to sing – and learn how to sing better. I had formal voice instruction in high school, with teachers who encouraged me to think about low breathing, deep breathing, and using my whole body when you breathe.

My first semester in college, I was so pleased when I found out about Yoga For Singers. We were doing a physical warm-up before our show, one that included yoga, and I overheard some of my cast mates discussing a yoga pose we were doing as one they had learned in the class. I made sure my advisor knew I wanted to take this class and signed up for it as soon as I could. I had practiced yoga in high school frequently and it was something that I had really enjoyed. One of my instructors, who had always stressed the rewards of physical activity as part of voice training, encouraged me to use yoga to help me with my breathing. Beyond making me feel more loose and relaxed in my body – which is really important for singers – yoga helps practitioners achieve a whole body experience. My voice teacher at college, Dr. Lister, also encouraged me to incorporate yoga into my routine as she knew all the issues I was having with breathing, such as building *sostenuto* strength and combating rib cage collapse at the ends of phrases.

To be very specific, there are a few poses like Up Dog, Side Angle and Triangle that specifically helped me to get my ribs more open. One of my main issues had been keeping them open at all times. Perfecting that through yoga practice has really helped me when I'm singing. I strive for that feeling that I have when I'm in yoga class

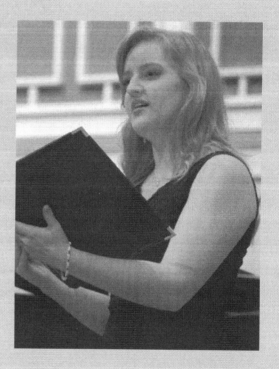

doing those poses, and it really helps me feel much more open and free.

I was able to experiment with yoga techniques on my own as well, and developed poses that worked for me and my breathing. The synergy between my YFS classes and my private voice instruction was really neat, though: during YFS class, there were times when my teacher would announce to the class, "This pose will help open up your ribs," and then she would look over at me with a smile on her face. It is this whole-body, organic approach to singing that I have found to be so rewarding, and I feel that yoga has not only brought balance to my voice, but also further enhanced it.

*–Emily Tweedy, voice performance major*

# Breathing Techniques

Pranayama is comprised of a number of different breathing techniques, many of which prove incredibly useful and are very applicable to singing. There is one feature of pranayama technique which we will avoid. Iyengar discusses the art of kumbhaka, or holding the breath between inhalation and exhalation. While this technique does indeed help to bring energy to the body and is based on centuries of tradition and practice, the practice of holding your breath can actually be counterproductive for singers. Unlike that of swimmers, the breath cycle of a singer should not include a holding period because it will most likely cause the support muscles to grab or lock and thus will impede the flow of the breath cycle. Holding their breath may make swimmers more buoyant in the water but it may make singers more rigid and thus can actually inhibit the buoyancy and resilience of their body. The dynamic resistance necessary for good *appoggio* or breath support is the antithesis of the swimmer's breath cycle since singers don't want to hold their breath and not breathe. Singing is pitched exhalation, so they have to use air but they want to control and extend their exhalation so that they can control their vocal phrasing.

In addition to incorporating awareness of the breath cycle by practicing breath-synchronized vinyasas, Iyengar stresses taking time to focus single-minded breath work without poses. Pranayama practice can be helpful before and/or after meditation but it requires focused, conscious respiration and should not incorporate other meditative methods. Pranayama is usually done in a seated position, either in Hero, Bound Angle, or Lotus position. Iyengar advises that "for the practice of pranayama there are two essentials: a stable (achala) spine, and a still (sthira) but alert mind."[6] To achieve these essential prerequisites, use some spine-lengthening asanas to elongate and stabilize the spine, then employ some balancing poses to center the mind. (Meditation can also help you find your focus, as will be discussed in Chapter Four, so meditation can be used before as well as after your pranayama practice.) When you have established these two conditions, then you are ready to begin work on the breathing techniques of pranayama.

*"Yoga composes my mind; it gives me more energy. As a singer, I also think some aspects of yoga, such as breathing properly, are key to maintaining a healthy voice. My lung capacity has also increased. I can certainly hold notes longer than I used to be able to do."*

—**Sting**, *rock singer, Yoga Journal, March 2010*

## KALA BREATH

Also known as Sufi mother's breath, the Kala (timed) breath involves establishing an equal ratio of inhalation and exhalation. Thus it focuses on equalizing the breath cycle and creating symmetry to the flow of the prana or energy.

- Inhale to a count of 4 and then exhale to a count of 4.
- You can either maintain the rhythmic flow of the cycle by repeating the 4-4 pattern or you can gradually increase the duration of counting.
- Just make sure that you don't start holding your breath in the inhalation stage and that the lungs do not start to feel "crowded."

Most of us are able to extend the duration of the exhalation much more easily than the duration of the inhalation, so I recommend not going above a count of 10. Even though some long vocal lines may last longer than 10 counts (for instance in Handelian or *bel canto* cadenzas), it is unlikely that the singer will have 10 counts to inhale. In addition to encouraging a long, slow inhalation, Sufi mother's breath calms the nervous system and energizes the respiratory organs. Use it to bring a sense of balance to your breath cycle and a steadiness to your psyche.

## UJJAYI BREATH

The relaxing and restorative Ujjayi breath is sometimes known as ocean breath, victorious breath, or sounding breath, but my class likes to call it the Darth Vader breath.

• First inhale slowly and deeply through the nose.
• As you exhale with a closed mouth and a closed glottis, engage the throat to form a narrow, focused path for the air as if you were making a whispering [hu] sound with a long, focused vocal tract.
• If you are having trouble, first try exhaling *bocca aperta* (with an open mouth) and imagine you are trying to fog up a mirror.
• Once you have the correct position then return to *bocca chiusa* (with a closed mouth).

When done properly the sound resembles the gentle roar of ocean waves or the iconic exhalation of the infamous *Star Wars* villain. According to Iyengar, Ujjayi breathing has remarkable, clarifying benefits for the singer:

> *This pranayama aerates the lungs, soothes and tones the nervous system. As a result of the deep respiratory action, the blood carries the supply of life-giving energy to the minutest parts of the tissues. It reduces phlegm, relieves pain in the chest, and the voice becomes melodious.*[7]

You can use the Ujjayi breath to slow down a rapid pulse and to deepen shallow breathing since it focuses the breath into a long, thin air stream, not unlike that used in good singing. In addition to focusing and slowing the exhalation, the Ujjayi breath focuses the mind, bringing a sense of calm centeredness. Thus, it can help relieve both physical and mental anxiety. I find it useful to do backstage before entering for a recital or opera role so that I can feel more serene and in control. An additional benefit of the Ujjayi breath, to which Iyengar alluded, is that it can gently shake phlegm off the cords without the negative effects of throat clearing. Enjoy the many rewards that the Ujjayi breath provides to both mind and body.

*"I do find that yoga is a great resource for me… a very calming, invigorating and challenging thing that I can do anywhere for my mental and physical health."*

—*Joyce Di Donato*, *mezzo-soprano, SFist interview, November 2009*

## ALTERNATE NOSTRIL BREATHING

The practice of alternate nostril breathing, also referred to as *nadi sodhana* or *anuloma viloma*, takes some getting used to but it is worth exploring.

• Before beginning your practice, be sure to wash your hands. This practice is not recommended if you are suffering from nasal congestion of any type, for obvious reasons!
• Close the right nostril with the right thumb and inhale through the left nostril.
• Release the thumb.
• Then close the left nostril with the right ring and pinkie fingers and exhale through the right nostril.
• Inhale through the right nostril and repeat the sequence, exhaling and then inhaling through the left nostril.

This pranayama technique has a noteworthy effect on focus and concentration, centering the mind in calm stillness. Furthermore, it is thought to balance and integrate the hemispheres of the brain. This aligning of brain hemispheres can be very advantageous to singers, who need to utilize the right brain to realize an intuitive, inspired, and risk-taking performance while the linear, logical left brain helps them to remember their lyrics and/or staging. Use this pranayama technique for balancing both the brain and the breath.

# BREATH OF FIRE

This vitalizing and cleansing breath is known by a number of names from the Skull Shining breath to *Kapalabhati*. A milder form of the Bellows Breath, it involves repeated exhilarating exhalations to energize the breath and body.

• Inhale through the nose.
• Then contract the abdomen inwards 10 times in quick pulses as if doing a series of *staccati* exhaling through the mouth.
• You may exhale in a succession of hissing sounds or imagine you are blowing out ten birthday candles.
• Inhale and exhale normally and then repeat.
• Keep the chest and shoulders still as you focus on working the abdominal muscles.

The Breath of Fire is especially useful if you are feeling lethargic or under-vitalized since it gets the blood and breath flowing quickly and creates heat and thus energy in the body. Furthermore, the Breath of Fire also helps cleanse the sinuses and is believed to help detoxify the lungs. Avoid this pranayama technique if you are pregnant, prone to fainting and lightheadedness, or if you have a hernia or high blood pressure. (In the 2008 *Incredible Hulk* movie, Edward Norton's character employed the Breath of Fire in an attempt to control his rage. But the Breathe of Fire would certainly elevate his heart rate, so he should have tried Kala or Ujjayi breathing instead!) The Breath of Fire should be enlivening and spine-tingling without being heady or breathtaking. It should bring buoyancy and freedom to staccato singing, enhancing coloratura arias such as Adele's Laughing Song in *Die Fledermaus* and Mabel's mirthful waltz "Poor Wandering One" from Gilbert and Sullivan's *The Pirates of Penzance*.

*"At one time I went on a lot of diets but just couldn't lose any weight. Then along came yoga and look at me now."*

—**Robert Merrill**, *Metropolitan Opera baritone, became a yoga devotee in the 1950s after it helped him lose twenty pounds. He was also fond of alternate nostril breathing, demonstrating the technique to reporters while sitting in Lotus position.*

*"I am into yoga, which is very stimulating. Very much into my yoga, very much into keeping my voice in its best shape as possible so that I would not do the unpardonable sin and cancel, or to be disappointing at all. Knowng this psychologically usually works."*

—**Leontyne Price**, *soprano, 1981 WTTW-TV interview*

## BELLOWS BREATH

If you found the Breath of Fire invigorating, then you may want to take it a step further with the Bellows Breath. This Kundalini pranayama technique called *Bhastrika* is an advanced breathing method that really stokes the fire, so it's not for everyone. It involves much more sharp and deliberate exhalations than the milder *Kapalabhati* breath. As Iyengar explains:

*In all other types of pranayama, inhalation sets the pace, the pattern, and the rhythm for exhalation. But in Bhastrika, exhalation sets the force and the pace. Here both out and in-breaths are vigorous and forceful. The sound is like that made by a blacksmith's bellows... Air is forcibly drawn in and out or blasted like a furnace.*[8]

- Begin with 5 rapid exhalations/expulsions and build up to 10 as you stoke the fire of your breath.
- You should feel your breath mechanism being heartily vitalized as heat and energy is rapidly created in your body.
- In addition, pay attention to the action and reaction of your rib and abdominal muscles.
- Feel them expand and contract quickly.
- Conclude your practice with slow inhalations before standing up in order to prevent dizziness or hyperventilation.

*"There is an amazing parallel [between yoga and singing]. When I sing, that's the other place where I feel utterly and completely in the moment. Both yoga and singing sort of bring me to that place. Five minutes before I go onstage, I do my pranayama."*

—**Sarah McLachlan**, *singer/songwriter, Yoga Journal, September 2010*

Because Bellows breathing is a more intense version of the Breath of Fire, it will have more intense effects on increasing circulation and oxygenation. Think of it as a Red Bull for respiration! Also, it has a heightened ability to clear the nasal passages, so be sure to have a box of Kleenex close at hand. Be careful with this powerful pranayama technique but if you choose to practice it, you will find a highly stimulating way to bring energy and elasticity to your abdominal breathing. Bellows breathing can also shed light on the panicked breathing of stage fright, since its rapid breath cycle might seem to mimic the quick breathing of anxiety. Instead, the Bellows Breath could be practiced in a gradual deceleration or *ritardando*. Then when the singer is confronted with brisk, anxious breathing they can use a Braking Bellows Breath to slow down the tempo of their breath cycle and bring it to a more manageable pace.

## SHITALI BREATH

If you feel overheated by stress or by doing the Breath of Fire or Bellows Breathing, then try this cooling pranayama technique. (It is usually done with the eyes closed, perhaps to prevent people from feeling self-conscious.)

• Roll the tongue, not in an Italian trilled r, but into a tube.

• Maintain your tongue position while you inhale and exhale through the mouth.

• If you don't have the genetic predisposition to roll the tongue in this way, then simply stick it out as if you are doing Lion pose. (For more on Lion pose, please see Chapter Three, page 81.)

• If you have a dog, he/she will show the perfect form for Shitali in his/her daily panting practice.

• Or you can do it with your mouth in the shape of an [o].

When performed with a rolled tongue, Shitali is believed to help quench thirst by stimulating the salivary glands. Therefore it can be a helpful tool in alleviating a nervous singer's dry mouth when no water is readily available. Think of Shitali as the pranayama of hypoventilation, therefore it makes an ideal cool-down after an intense pranayama workout.

Practice these pranayama exercises as a way to improve your breath support for singing and your breath control for stress management. Remember that prana is life, so breathe to live (and sing) well instead of live to breathe.

# EVERY BREATH YOU TAKE: MUSIC FOR PRANAYAMA PRACTICE

For practicing the measured breathing of Kala breath, it is important to inhale and exhale to a symmetrical count. (For example, inhale for 4 beats, exhale for 4 beats.) It can help to practice breathing to a song about breathing! Here is a lengthy list of artists from differing genres with songs bearing the title, "**Breathe.**"

- Faith Hill
- Anna Nalick
- Michelle Branch
- Taylor Swift
- Melissa Ethridge
- U2
- Jill Scott
- Michael W. Smith
- Depeche Mode
- Collective Soul
- Erasure
- plus the *In the Heights* Broadway soundtrack

R & B singer Toni Braxton has a number of songs on the subject ("**Breathe Again**" and "**I'm Still Breathing**"). Considering its focus on medical (and emotional) trauma, I suppose it makes sense that the popular television drama *Grey's Anatomy* also features many songs about remembering to breathe. Their soundtracks have included "**Breathe In, Breathe Out**" by Mat Kearney and the mantra-like "**Keep Breathing**" by Ingrid Michaelson.

If you prefer to practice your pranayama to classical music, there are numerous art songs about breathing ("**Lasciami! Lascia ch'io respiri/Let me breathe**" by Francesco Tosti) and sighing (Henri Duparc's "**Soupir**"). In addition, there are soothing Mozart opera excerpts about the flowing movement of air which are highly applicable to the breath cycle such as "**Sull'aria/ Che soave zeffiretto**" (On the air/What a gentle breeze), duet from *Le nozze di Figaro*, and "**Soave sia il vento**" (Gentle is the wind), trio from *Così fan tutte*. The Figaro duet played a prominent part in the award-winning film *The Shawshank Redemption* (1994), while both Mozart ensembles are found on the Philips CD *More Mozart for Mothers-to-Be*.

# 3

## Asanas for Alignment

*"Asanas bring health, beauty, strength, firmness, lightness, clarity of speech and expression, calmness of the nerves and a happy disposition."*

—B.K.S. Iyengar

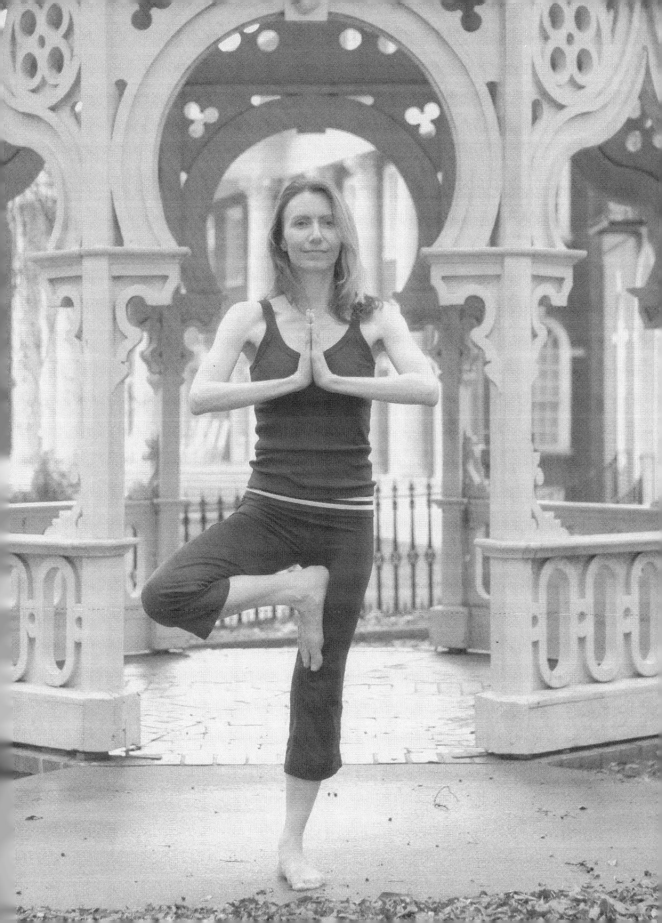

In Iyengar's description, asanas are the perfect prescription for all ills! Although they may not be a panacea, asanas can definitely serve a number of useful purposes for singers. Above all, asanas have a profoundly positive effect on proper posture or alignment. In the apt words of opera director Mark Ross Clark, "Alignment is not solely for an aesthetic look of strength for the singing actor; it is imperative for free vocal production and freedom of movement."[9] The singer's instrument is his body and ideal alignment of the instrument enhances and enables optimal vocal technique and thereby empowers healthy, and heartfelt, singing.

## CELEBRITY YOGIS:

Reportedly, yoga has been part of the pre-performance regimes of Broadway musical stars **Betty Buckley** and **Sutton Foster**, country singers **LeAnn Rimes**, **Kenny Chesney** and **Taylor Swift**, *Glee* star **Lea Michele**, self-described "classical pop singer" **Sarah Brightman**, verismo opera diva **Magda Olivero**, Latin pop singer **Ricky Martin**, and hip-hop artist/vegan **André 3000** (formerly of OutKast)

Asana means "seat" in Sanskrit and this term is used to describe the physical positions or poses of hatha yoga. Iyengar yoga places particular emphasis on alignment and posture in the asanas. There is no perfect yoga posture, no perfect pose in that no one's body is "perfect." Since we are neither clones nor machines, we each possess a unique instrument. We must be aware of the strengths and weaknesses of our own body just as we need to know the unique assets and challenges our singing voices possess. "Perfection" in every yoga posture is an unattainable goal, but proper alignment in the poses is absolutely necessary, not for reasons of aesthetics or vanity but for health and safety. Improper form could lead to injury, while ideal postural alignment allows you to fully realize the manifold benefits of the poses. So while there is no perfect pose, a properly performed pose will nurture healthy alignment and ideal muscular coordination so that singers can train their muscles to achieve proper alignment off the yoga mat and onstage. To help achieve this goal of proper alignment, Iyengar introduced the use of props to help students to find good form while progressing in their practice of the poses. By using yoga blocks and/or straps, you can enjoy the benefits of the asanas even if you cannot yet achieve the ultimate version of the asana. Usually nine inches long, six inches wide and four inches tall, a yoga block is simply a foam or wooden block useful in modifying poses to one's current flexibility or providing support in maintaining asanas. Similarly, a yoga strap is a cotton (or sometimes hemp) strap used in stretching poses to increase flexibility without strain or injury. For instance, the strap should loop around the balls of your feet in a seated forward bend if you cannot yet touch your toes. One could also use a resistance band or even a piece of elastic. These yoga props add stability and security, especially to a beginning practitioner, by making poses more reachable, nurturing balance, and aiding in alignment. A new product called Yoga-Paws can also be helpful for those traveling without a yoga mat. These toe socks and half-gloves are like mini yoga mats for your hands and feet which can help you from slipping when practicing Downward-Facing Dog in your room at the Hyatt.[a]

*"For a singer, to sing with poor posture... limits the instrument. Many students haven't thought in terms of the whole body as the instrument. Postural work can be gained from more than just the voice teacher... Yoga is good for mind/body centering."*

—**Carol Webber**, *Professor of Music, Eastman School of Music (and my former teacher)*

---

a  Yoga-Paws ([www.yogapaws.com](www.yogapaws.com)) are highly portable but are not recommended for Bikram yoga and should be removed for proper practice of the mudras or hand yoga postures. (See Chapter 4.)

# YOGA: IT'S NOT JUST FOR SKINNY PEOPLE!

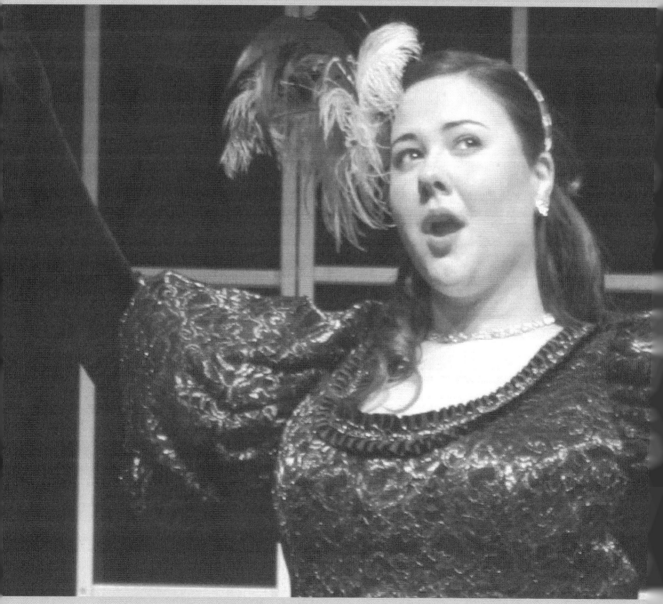

Laura Collins, B.M. in voice performance

I'm flexible despite the fact that I'm overweight, as are a lot of people who may be beyond their ideal body weight. And the great thing about yoga – which was really pushed in the Yoga For Singers class – is it's not about what you can or can't do when you start, it's about how far you can go during the journey. For someone like me, who doesn't have the body type one stereotypically correlates with yoga, such a class outlook has helped me to both realize my limitations and give me a chance to grow.

There were a few poses that presented difficulties due to my weight, mainly ones where I have to hold myself up with my hands. I would feel a bit limited with those (like Crow, for example), but I quickly learned that if you can't do the pose because of size or injury, there's always going to be an alternative pose that will be just as effective as the one you can't do.

Another example might be Wheel, where one does a backbend like one might do in gymnastics. Not ideal for me! But the purpose of that pose is to help lengthen the spine, so an alternate for Wheel would be Fish, which helps in both lengthening the spine and elevating the sternum. It helps with breath support and enables me to feel more grounded when I perform, a fantastic option when I need to feel the length in my body so I can get long, low breaths.

Before entering the YFS class, it's not like I was intimidated because it was something I didn't think I could do. Once I got in the class, I quickly proved that to myself. There was, however, dealing with the idea that I most definitely did not fit the general stereotype of "yoga practitioner as stick figure." I was worried that I'd look foolish and out of place, even though I knew I could cut it physically. But I got over that soon enough, and I never felt neurotic about things unless I accidentally wore clothing that made me feel vulnerable. The reason why is our instructor created the kind of classroom setting where I knew my contribution was just as valid as anyone else's. That definitely put me at ease. In fact, none of my overweight peers ever expressed any concerns that I was aware of. There were girls in the class that were twice my size, and they never seemed to feel inadequate or made fun of, simply because we were all there and all trying to see how far we could progress. Nobody was judging anyone else based on what they could or couldn't do. Our YFS teacher did a good job making us feel good about not obsessing over how we looked with each pose – not, "Oh my gosh, my pants are so tight!"

It doesn't matter what size you are – as long as you are able to find the perfect pose within yourself, you can achieve what the pose was meant to do! Some starter poses I would recommend for overweight practitioners include the Sun Salutation; that whole vinyasa – Mountain-dive into Plank-Up Dog-Down Dog – is fantastic. Also, Bridge really challenges all aspects of your body, especially the spine – it's user-friendly and very easy, because it helps you become aware of your spine as you roll through the vertebrae.

The upshot for me in doing yoga is that it helps me feel at home in my body not alien to my body. That physical component of yoga then blends into a positive mental state of being, bringing with it a calming effect and a good way of finding a center. It doesn't matter whether you're skinny or overweight, or man or woman, whenever we talk about "body image," what that really translates to is, "How do I look?" Obsessing over that can be a real deterrent to everyday mental stability, so yoga has a real use in helping people find a center that connects your present day physical being with your feelings of self-worth and self-image.

You know how it's always said that, in opera, "It ain't over 'til the fat lady sings." If it's me you're talking about, just imagine that "fat lady" doing yoga warm-ups before she goes on stage to hit that high note! [Author's Note: The ever humble Miss Collins is not a fat lady!]

ASSOCIATION OF SINGERS WHO HATE YOGA:

*"A group for singers who are sick and tired of being told how great yoga is for your posture, breathing, singing, stage presence, blah blah blah blah.... If you've done one too many downward dogs, if plank pose makes you grouchy, if you'd rather salute the sun with your middle finger, then this group is for you."*

—*Facebook group, 4 members*

*Yes, voice students may tire of hearing their teachers' repeated advice, and yoga is not for everyone, but this group's small contingent may not have had a yoga class which helped them fully appreciate the connection between yoga and singing. Or maybe they should try kickboxing.*

Most singers know the elements of good postural alignment, no doubt because their voice teachers have made repeated references to it. Postural work is primary in beginning voice instruction and remains an important concept. In fact, while voice teachers notoriously disagree on certain things, there is little argument that healthy and proper posture assists healthy and proper breathing. The singer should strive for an elevated or "noble" chest, a wide rib cage and a long, aligned spine. The shoulders should not be raised but rolled slightly backwards to assist the lengthening of the spine, on which the neck and head should rest freely. Although many singers may be able to describe proper posture, approximating it can be a much more challenging endeavor. In fact, many singers inadvertently create deleterious muscular tension in their well-intentioned attempts at creating and/or maintaining good alignment. Vocal pedagogue James McKinney insightfully observes that this type of "tension probably is the greatest enemy of the public performer" since "good posture precedes good breathing"[10] and good singing, and improper alignment impedes all three.

Iyengar emphasized the sequencing of the asanas into a flow or vinyasa. Meaning "to place in a certain way," a vinyasa is a specific sequence of poses which flow together synchronizing movement of the body with the breath. The sequence of poses could be a traditional one such as a Sun Salutation (12 asanas performed in order in a series) or a vinyasa designed with particular emphasis on specific body parts (i.e. spine, ribs, hips). The sequence of asansas trains the body to find its

*"It's easy to go through the day and not observe one's own consciousness and patterns of thought. I find that the act of doing yoga prepares me to meditate. I'm forced to slow down, observe my body and mind. By working on my body, it gets easier; I feel more in tune with my emotions."*

*—**Daniel Okulitch**, bass-baritone, used yoga to prepare for the physically demanding title role in the premiere of L.A. Opera's "The Fly" (based on the classic film and conducted by famed tenor Placido Domingo).*

ideal alignment and helps to create muscle memory of that good posture which can be taken into your daily life. Reliable vocal technique is all about muscle memory, and it is easier for your muscles to remember how they should be helping you stand well when you sing if it is the same way that you stand on a regular, everyday basis. In addition, the concept of breathing through the sequence of poses has two benefits for singers. First, it reinforces a concept of the breath cycle, which is one of the primary principles of good vocal technique. Secondly, breathing through the challenges and stretches of yoga poses encourages the singer to breathe through physical and emotional challenges, a useful approach in dealing with the stresses of performance anxiety and stage fright.

DIVA DESSAY'S ADVICE
TO YOUNG SINGERS:

*"Have acting lessons. Yoga or dance, or something with your body. I just started yoga. And I like it very much. I really decided that I'm going to have [yoga] lessons on a regular basis, and steady basis, as much as possible."*

—**Natalie Dessay**, *Classical Singer Magazine, September 2009*

Asanas assist in developing body awareness, which will help singers' physical presence onstage, whether they have to dance (like Masetto and Zerlina at their wedding in *Don Giovanni*) or sing while lying in bed during a dramatic death scene (à la Mimi, Violetta, et al). It is surprisingly difficult to sing well in an operatic death scene, because sitting up in bed while pretending to die of tuberculosis is not conducive to good singing. Dying onstage takes a lot of abdominal awareness in order to sing your character's last notes with haunting beauty. In an incredibly impressive display of abdominal core strength and excellent spinal alignment, soprano Natalie Dessay sang a high Eb while being carried offstage in a horizontal position in Laurent Pelly's 2008 Metropolitan Opera production of *La Fille du Régiment*. Balancing poses may prove especially difficult at times but they have measurable benefits in focus and concentration, important skills for singers as they prepare for a performance. Alignment and balance are both important for the singer playing Porgy in *Porgy and Bess*, not to mention good knees since he must sing the entire opera while kneeling. The title role of *Rigoletto* also provides postural challenges since it requires portraying a hunchbacked jester without sacrificing necessary alignment for singing. In fact, singers playing a variety of character parts and/or older characters (i.e. Billy's grandmother in *Billy Elliot* or Grandpa Joe in *Willy Wonka*) might be directed to round the spine, so they need the awareness and ability to portray such characters' physicality without harming their spine or hindering their singing.

There are literally millions of asanas (8,400,000 according to ancient yogic scriptures) but some of particular relevance to singers will be the focus of this chapter. These apt asanas include those which help lengthen the spine, open the ribs, relax shoulder tension, and free the neck. Although headstands are a valid component of many schools of yoga, they will be avoided in the suggested vinyasas along with other neck-compressing postures which could put pressure on the larynx. To sing healthfully, there should be no tension in the neck area, and it is very difficult to do headstands correctly and avoid having both gravity and the weight of the entire body pressing down on the head and neck (and the larynx). Headstands and handstands can be intimidating and frightening even to seasoned yoga practitioners, so we will avoid them here to avoid pressure on the neck and to keep the asanas accessible and non-threatening.

You will notice that the asanas are often named after flora and fauna. Those singers who are accustomed to holistic voice teachers or the use of imagery in their lessons will find the asanas' names helpful in achieving the pose, imagining they are the animal or the object they are emulating. Naming the yoga pose after a cow, a giraffe or a dolphin helps bring a role-playing element to yoga practice, something that suits most singers' theatrical personalities. Plus the imagery simply makes the poses more imaginative and fun.

Before you begin your asana practice, get ready to throw some ego and insecurity out the window. As with singing, practicing yoga requires that you relinquish a certain amount of vanity. For instance a good singing breath demands an expansion in the lower abdomen. If you are self-conscious or worried about looking fat, then you won't be able to let this expansion take place fully and thus you won't be able to breathe as well. When trying the asanas, you need to not worry about looking "funny" or "stupid" and embrace the absurdity (and fun!) of poses named after animals. If you don't give the poses a chance, then you won't be able to enjoy their benefits for your body and your voice. Don't let angst about your size prevent you from doing a pose either: no one is calling you a fat cow in Cow pose! Of course we all have physical limitations, and you want to be aware of them and careful of them. For example, if you had scoliosis and had a rod put in your spine, then arching you back into Cow pose may not be possible. Recognize any legitimate medical conditions or concerns (joint or back problems, heart issues, pregnancy,[b] previous injuries, etc) but don't

---

b There are many outlets for Pre-Natal Yoga, which is designed protect the baby while helping prepare mom for birth.

JENNIFER LOPEZ
IS ANOTHER YOGA
CONVERT:

*"When I was younger, I was into hard physical exercise, but now what's more important to me is finding a balance of mind, body and spirit."*

—*Jennifer Lopez*

let them add perceived limitations to your practice. With both singing and doing yoga, worrying about "looking good" prevents you from doing your best. Worrying about how the class or the audience thinks you look distracts you from staying focused on your form, technique, craft, and art and can even feed your performance anxiety. Focus on the pose at hand and you will free your mind from distraction and grant your body greater freedom and better form.

The old "no pain, no gain" mentality common in some sports is not compatible with yoga practice. There will be mild discomfort in stretching if you want to increase your flexibility and go further in the poses, but you should never push yourself to "feel the burn" or you might feel yourself pulling a muscle. Try to relax into the stretch by using your exhalation to help your muscles release deeper into the position. Always listen carefully to your body and err on the side of caution. Yoga is not about competition or getting there <u>now</u>, it is an ongoing journey. Enjoy the process of yoga practice just like a singer must enjoy practicing because one will be (or should be!) practicing more than one is performing. Remember to be aware of any personal medical issues which may impact your practice, but explore the asanas with an open mind (and body) without feeling like you have something to prove. As I tell my students, there is no yoga event in the Olympics (although Ashtanga yoga became a demonstration sport at the 2008 games in Beijing and there is an underground movement, going against yoga's origins, lobbying for yoga to become a competitive sport). Yoga is not meant to be a strength contest or flexibility face-off with others so you shouldn't push beyond your limits. Instead, explore the poses and try to go deeper into each pose but only to the point where you are challenged.

# Basic Starting Asanas

Once you are doing vinyasas and meditation, these poses are where you will often begin (Mountain, Staff) and end (Lotus, Corpse).

## MOUNTAIN

A seemingly simple pose of obvious relevance to singers as they stand in the nook of the piano at a performance or audition. Also the starting point for most standing poses and vinyasas, this asana invokes positive physical imagery of tall stature, as well as positive mental imagery of reaching the summit in your singing.

Stand tall with your feet parallel, hip-width apart. Shoulders are rolled down and back, and arms hang freely at your sides. Balance your weight evenly on your feet and focus on lining up the ankles, hips, shoulders, neck, and head. You should feel like your body is one tall, strong unit ascending to its zenith. Try to open the chest but be careful not to sway or arch the back.

For Tall Mountain pose, simply raise the arms straight overhead, keeping the palms facing inward. (To deepen the pose, bring the palms together in this straight-arm, overhead position.). Make sure the shoulders stay down while your arms reach to the sky along with your tall spine.

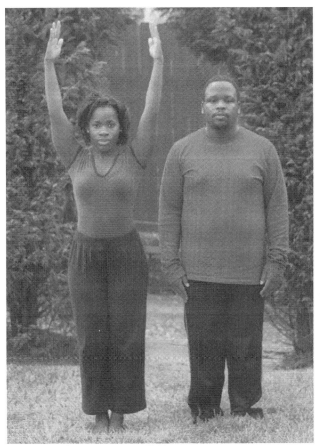

Tall Mountain (left) and Mountain pose (right).
"Climb Ev'ry Mountain."—Rodgers and Hammerstein's *The Sound of Music*

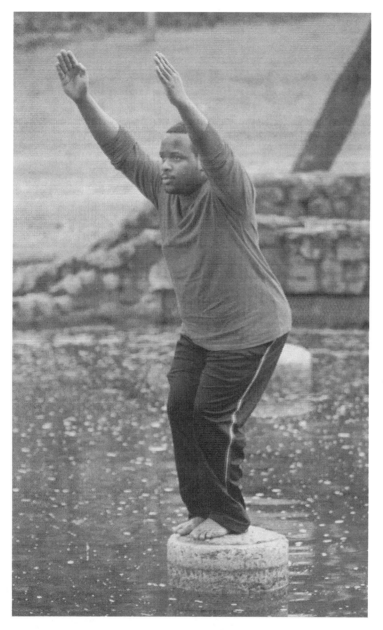

## CHAIR

An excellent leg strength-ener, Chair quickly cre-ates vitality in the body. It builds leg strength so you can stand onstage with greater presence and solidity.

From Tall Mountain, bend the knees as if you were sitting back into a chair. Be sure to keep the knees together and the shoulders down. The back should arch a bit and you should avoid leaning forward or collapsing the chest. This asana makes me think of "Sit Down, You're Rocking the Boat" from *Guys and Dolls*.

"In my own little corner, in my own little chair." –more Rodgers & Hammerstein, *Cinderella*

## STAFF AND L POSE

**Staff** is a starting point for seated vinyasas.

Sit with your legs together extended in front of your torso with feet flexed. Strive for a long, extended spine, reaching tall like a staff of wheat, as you let your palms rest at your sides or on the floor. Without arching the back, feel the front of the spine lengthening as you reach the sternum towards the ceiling. This pose will help greatly with learning to sit well and combat slouching, important when stage blocking requires you to sit and sing consumptive death scenes like in *La Traviata*! It is also helpful for voice teachers, who spend their days sitting on the piano bench.

**L Pose** is a physical enactment of the letter L.

Think of it as a dorsal version of Staff pose. It helps blood circulate to the brain, increasing mental acuity and focus, thereby keeping the mind sharp and song lyrics more easily recalled on command. Lie on your back and extend the legs upwards at a ninety-degree angle. Keep the feet flexed and rest the arms palms down on the floor next to your torso. Or try doing it by lying on your back with your buttocks against a wall, running your legs upwards along a wall. L pose is especially helpful after a long period of standing onstage, as during a long song cycle such as *Die Winterreise*.

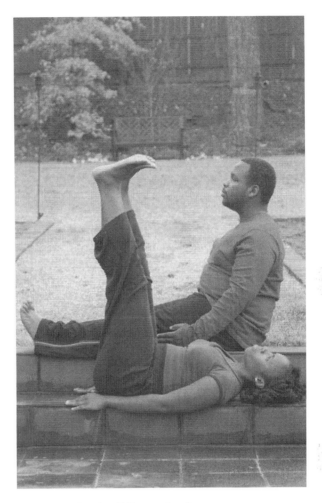

Staff (background pose) and L (foreground pose)

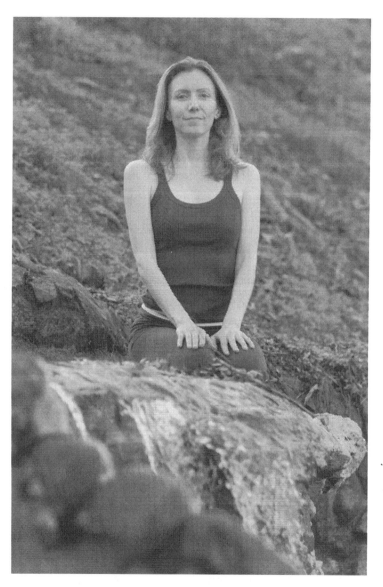

"I Need a Hero." –from *Footloose* (and *Shrek 2*)

## HERO

Sometimes called Thunderbolt, it helps you maintain a feeling of power in the body even though it is a seated pose.

Kneel on the floor with your knees together then sit back, resting your buttocks on your heels while you sit up straight and extend the spine. Rest the palms on the thighs. Use a blanket for support under your knees if you need, or sit on a block (or two). As with Staff pose, think of a high, noble chest so desirous in singers and feel the front of your body lengthening and opening. An obligatory pose for anyone playing *Madama Butterfly* or *Miss Saigon*, Hero is believed to help the symptoms of asthma.

# BOUND ANGLE

Also known as Butterfly, it nurtures the singer's noble posture while seated, in addition to loosening the hips for freer movement onstage.

Start in Staff pose, then bend the knees and bring the soles of the feet together. Make sure the spine is long as you clasp the ankles with your hands. For an additional stretch in the hips and inner thighs, bring the feet closer towards the body as long as you don't strain the knees. Keep the chest lifted and enjoy the hip stretch of this pose. For a deeper stretch, you may extend the upper body out over the legs, trying to keep a long spine. Then for a counter stretch, round the spine and try to reach your forehead towards your feet or the floor. When done this way, you will get a wonderful stretch for both the front and back of your spine as well as the hips.

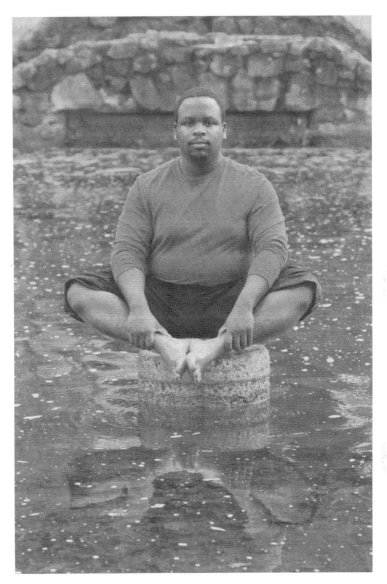

Country singer Shania Twain, a devotee of Sant Mat meditation, meditates in Bound Angle.

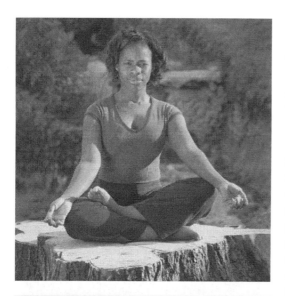

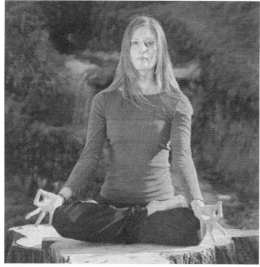

Half Lotus (top) and Full Lotus (bottom), as in Robert Schumann's "Die Lotosblume."

# HALF OR FULL LOTUS

The full traditional position for seated mudra meditation, most often done near the end of class. This pose is ideal for mantra meditation before a performance.

Sitting "Indian" style (Easy pose) with the right foot in front, lift the right foot and rest it gently on the thigh of the left leg. Try to keep the toes spread open like the petals of a blooming lotus flower. This is Half Lotus. To go into Full Lotus, maintain this position but move the left foot on top of the right thigh. Gently RR.[c] Be gentle with your knees and be patient with this pose. It should be a place where you can maintain good posture (tall spine, high sternum) while focusing your mind inward for meditation. Don't be frustrated if you can't do Full Lotus or if Half Lotus is a challenge. Work toward the pose's positive actions (calming the brain, enlivening the spine) and try meditating in Hero, Bound Angle or Easy Pose (Indian-style) instead if needed.

[c] RR=Release and repeat on the other side.

# CORPSE

Often the final pose of a yoga class, ideal for relaxation or mantra meditation before an audition, recital, or show.

Lie flat on your back, supine. Keep your hands at your sides with your palms facing upwards. Extend the legs along the floor keeping them slightly apart and letting the hips open and the feet roll outwards. Close your eyes and relax the entire body. For an additional release and spine stretch, have a partner or your teacher gently lift your legs a few inches and pull them away from the center of the body before setting them gently back on the floor. Have them repeat with the same sequence with your arms. Then have them gently lift your head off the ground as they support and gently lengthen the neck. This "adjustment" should leave your spine feeling luxuriously long and released. If your lower back still feels pressure or a bit of a sway or upward arch, hug the knees into the chest and then release the legs out long to rest in Corpse. Or you can use a blanket under your head or your knees to support them as needed. This restorative pose helps you release and realign so that you can arise from the asana with new-found vitality and serenity. It may also come in handy for lying still and controlling your breath while playing dead as Mimi in *La bohème* or Tony, Riff, and Bernardo in *West Side Story*.

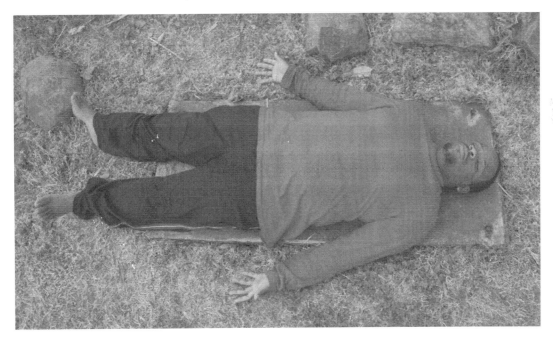

Meditate to Richard Strauss's *Tod und Verklärung* (Death and Transfiguration).

# Spine-lengthening Asanas

Lengthening the spine is integral and invaluable to maintaining good posture. Good posture helps you present yourself more confidently onstage (and helps you sing better). For instance, a singer who enters an audition with a tall, long spine projects poise, assurance, and even competence, while a slouched singer presents an impression of one who is meek in their confidence and perhaps even talent. When someone is called spineless, he/she is considered to be lacking in courage, guts, or grit. Yet all of these qualities are absolutely necessary for a performer, so you need to be full of spine! Most of all, poor posture is functionally inefficient because it inhibits good breathing by diminishing lung capacity and hindering physical freedom, and thereby good singing. So there are many reasons to work on lengthening the spine. Think of your spine as an extension of your unique brain. Your spinal cord is your means of taking thought from your brain into action by your body, so nurture this vital link between your artistic impulses and your vocal feats.

In the excellent *Yoga Journal* video *Yoga Practice for Flexibility*, yoga goddess/guru and Iyengar disciple (not to mention human pretzel) Patricia Walden inspires the viewer to think of his/her spine moving towards the head "like a free, flowing river."[1] This image is a great asset to the practice of these spine-lengthening asanas. In addition, it is helpful to imagine the concept of Kundalini energy uncoiling through your constantly elongating spinal column. Whenever you stretch, remember that it takes 30 seconds for a muscle being stretched to release, so hold any stretching poses for at least 30 seconds. Keep breathing through the stretch, inhaling as you lift a little and then exhaling as you press gently and try to take the stretch deeper.

# CHILD

A wonderful resting pose that opens the shoulders and calms the mind when performance nerves are unsettling.

Start kneeling with the knees hip-width apart. Sit back on your heels, trying to fold your upper body onto your thighs. Reach your arms out straight in front of you on the floor with palms facing downward and rest your forehead on the floor. Keep space between the fingers for an additional hand stretch. For more stretch in the shoulders, keep reaching the hands out farther away from the body as you sit back on your heels or widen the opening of the hips to bring your chest on the floor between your thighs. Alternately, you can bring the arms to rest on the floor next to your legs. With the palms upward, you should feel a stretch in the upper back as gravity widens the space between the shoulder blades. From this rejuvenating fetal position, you can find great stress relief and serenity.

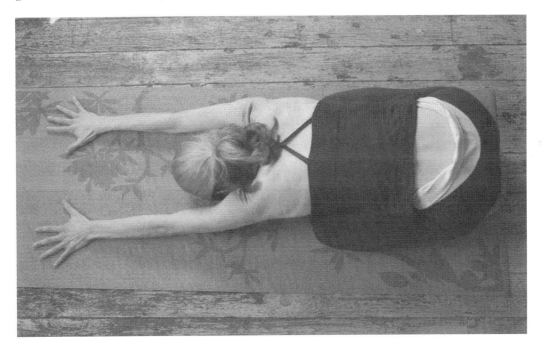

Imagine "The Children's Hour," the well-loved Charles Ives song.

## COW

A partner to Cat pose, it helps in lifting the sternum for the wide ribs needed for good breathing for singing.

From kneeling on all fours with a flat-back position, drop the belly and arch your back, looking upwards and lifting the chest as you inhale. You should feel a lengthening of the front of the spine. Doing Cat and Cow in tandem massages the spine both front and back and cultivates balance in the muscles of your back. It also helps build core strength if you utilize the abdominals to initiate the movement from Cow into Cat pose.

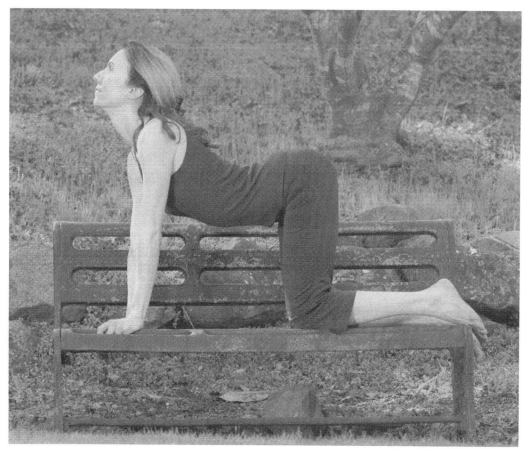

For calm before your cattle call audition.

# CAT

A luxurious spinal stretch, it helps release the shoulder tension so common in singers.

From Cow pose, exhale and engage the abdominals as you contract/ round your back upwards to the ceiling (or sky if outdoors!) like a cat awakening from a nap. You should feel a great broadening of the upper back and shoulders, space between the vertebrae, and a refreshing stretch of your spinal column. When I practice this pose at home, my cats always circle around my legs as if they are expressing approval of this feline-inspired asana.

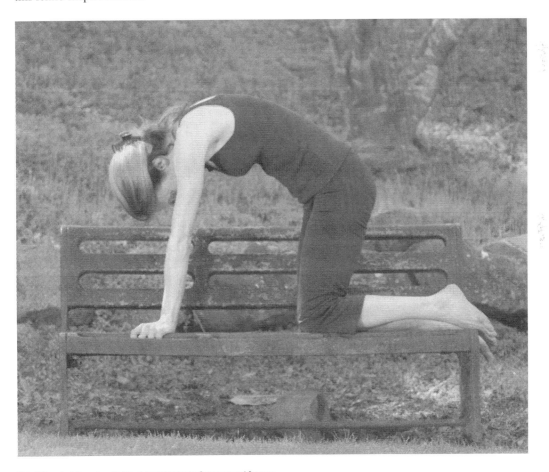

This feline stretch evokes Andrew Lloyd Webber's *Cats* now and forever.

## PLANK

The perfect push-up position.

Start lying prone, on your belly. Keeping the feet together and the hands directly under the shoulders, straighten your elbows and lift yourself into push-up position, making sure your body is in one straight line. Be sure to engage the abdomen to support the spine and make sure that the back does not arch in either direction. Most people will either let the hips sag towards the ground, or leave the hips too high so that their plank more closely resembles Downward-facing Dog pose. Plank makes you focus on aligning the spine while fighting the pull of gravity. It will help greatly with your kinesthetic sense of standing alignment which you can then take onstage.

Plank pose can help you achieve the impressive pectoral muscles of barihunks Keith Miller (professional football player turned Escamillo) or Rodney Gilfry (as Stanley Kowalski, Marlon Brando's role in André Previn's opera *A Streetcar Named Desire*).

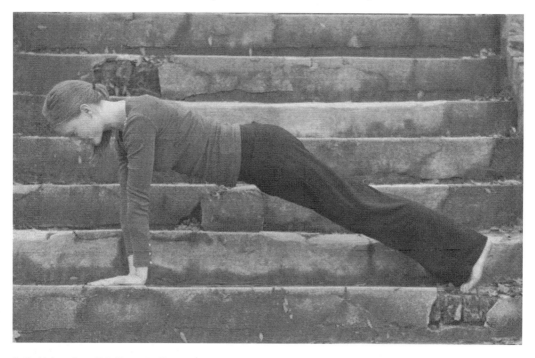

No Doubt singer Gwen Stefani is great at Plank pose.

# REVERSE PLANK

A challenging asana that again helps in lifting the sternum for great stage posture.

Start in Staff pose. With your hands (fingertips facing forward) next to your hips, straighten the arms and lift the hips off the floor until you are in a perfect reversal of push-up position. Again, be careful not to let the hips sag towards the ground. You could have a practice partner use a yoga strap under your hips to help pull them upwards. Besides helping with alignment, Reverse Plank also helps strengthen the position of the noble chest and stretches the front of the spine. A fringe benefit of Reverse Plank is toned triceps, so women can minimize what some refer to as "bat wings" and thereby feel confident wearing sleeveless gowns onstage.

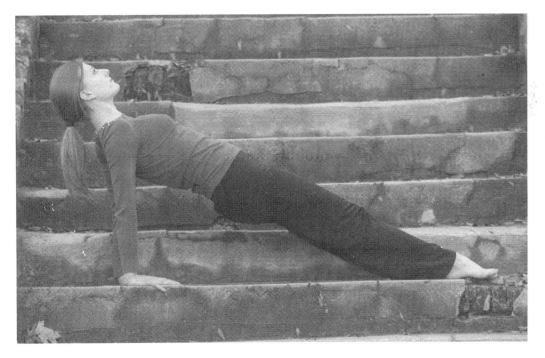

"I dare you to lift yourself up off the floor." –Switchfoot

## LOCUST

A lovely spine lengthener and another great sternum elevator for singers.

Lying prone with your arms at your sides, keep the legs together and straight as you lift them off the ground. Simultaneously lift the arms back straight towards the feet, palms facing upwards. Stretch the body long like a locust in flight. This pose will bolster back strength and help you stand up straight. Ladies, it will also make you look sleek and toned in your backless recital dress!

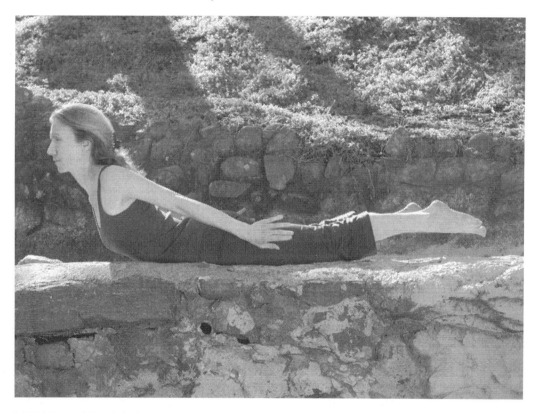

In Ernest Chausson's "Les cigales," the cicadas "sing better than the violins."

## BOW

A favorite of children, especially when they rock back and forth.

Lying on your stomach, bend the knees and reach back with the arms to grasp your ankles and lift yourself upwards. Try one leg at a time (Half Bow) if the back does not feel strong enough yet to sustain this intense arch. Really focus on rolling the shoulders back and lifting the chest so this pose can reinforce the noble posture of good singing. Bow pose strengthens the back muscles while stretching the front of the body, cultivating the high sternum and expanded ribs necessary for good breathing and good singing. You could also try Bow pose with a partner gently pulling back on your heels to help you lift the chest more and expand the rib cage.

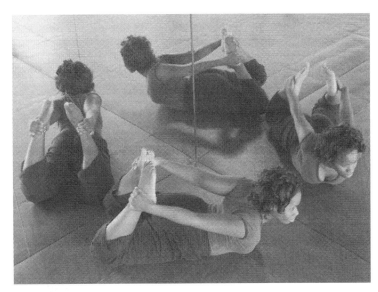

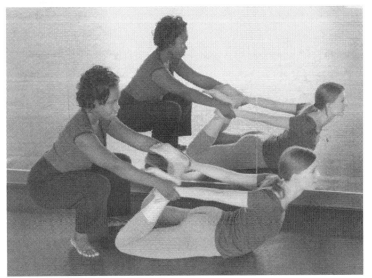

Coloratura Kristin Chenoweth has been seen *Glee*-fully performing Bow pose at NYC's Yogamaya studio.

## UPWARD-FACING DOG

A supreme spine strengthener, it helps singers learn to roll the shoulders back into proper placement. Just as Cow and Cat poses usually go together, Up Dog often precedes its canine counter pose, Down Dog.

From a prone position on your belly, place your hands on the floor right next to the rib cage and inhale as you straighten the arms to lift yourself upwards. Keeping the feet about a foot apart, make sure the shoulders press downwards as you stretch the arms, leg and spine. The tops of the feet remain on the floor while the hips lift off a bit (which helps distinguish Up Dog from Cobra pose). Arch the back and look upwards. Besides stretching and strengthening the spine, Up Dog braces the shoulder yoke and assists in optimal upper body alignment.

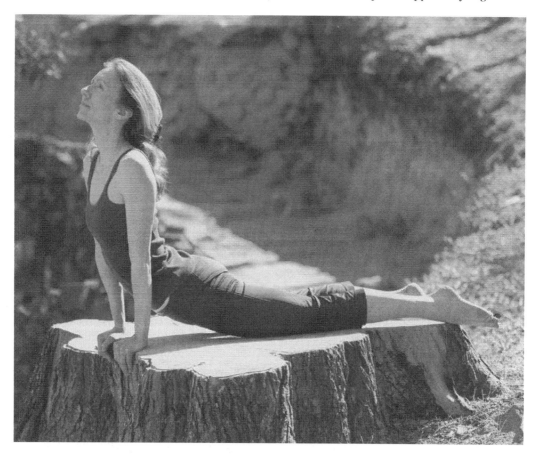

"Up-up-up-There's no way but up from here. " –Shania Twain

# DOWNWARD-FACING DOG

A great shoulder stretch and stress reliever, it is perhaps the best known asana and my personal favorite pre-singing pose.

Down Dog is usually approached from Up Dog. From Up Dog, lower yourself flat on your belly and curl the toes under so they are helping support you. Lifting your tailbone towards the ceiling, exhale and straighten the legs and arms so that your body makes an upside-down V-shape with your pelvis tilting upwards and your hips centered between your hands and feet. Keep the back flat instead of rounded and think of lifting your tailbone to the sky (or ceiling). The head should be in line with the arms so as not to strain the back of the neck or compress the larynx. Try to reach the heels towards the floor. In addition to its superlative stretch of the shoulders, Down Dog creates a sense of width and stability in the rib cage and torso. As long as they're still reaching, don't worry if your heels never reach the ground. If they do reach, then you might try lifting the toes for an additional/occasional variation on the stretch. Work hard on this pose until it feels familiar since it is such an important asana. It helps singers with building upper body strength, energizing the entire body, and calming the brain. It is even believed to have therapeutic effects on asthma and sinusitis. This is why I find it a wonderful asana for a backstage vinyasa (see vinyasa sequence later in the chapter).

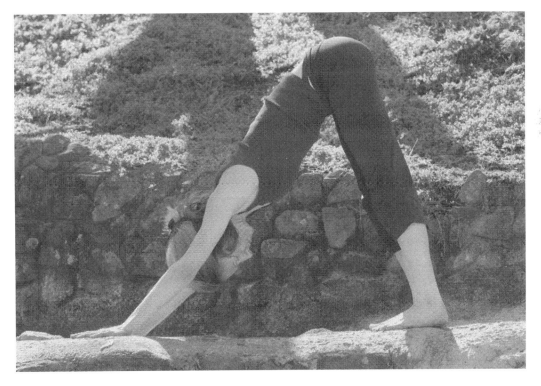

"Down to earth." –Peter Gabriel, *WALL-E*

# WARRIOR 3

A challenging table-top balance which, like Plank, creates awareness of alignment that can give you a taller presence onstage.

From Mountain pose, reach the arms overhead in Tall Mountain. Then simultaneously lift the working leg backwards as you balance on the standing leg, and lower the arms forward until both arms and the back leg are parallel to the floor. Stretch the body in one long line from fingertips to your big toe. RR. Warrior 3 should help spinal alignment and will empower you via its balancing challenge. For a different entry into Warrior 3, start in Mountain pose with hands at your sides, then lift the arms forward as your lift one leg backwards so your body makes a long warrior's spear shape from finger to toe. I tell my students to make their back nice and flat so that someone could have a tea party on it without spilling.

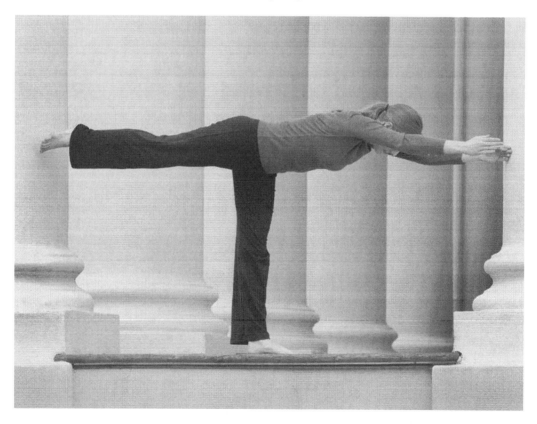

"Soldiers of Peace." –Crosby, Stills and Nash

# TREE

Always a class favorite, this balancing pose turns normally loquacious singers silent. Tree helps focus the mind and body, thus it helps bring focus to the performer in presenting and remembering text.

From Mountain pose, shift your weight to one foot and place the sole of the other foot on the calf or inner thigh of the standing leg. Press the foot into the leg in an isometric exercise. Avoid pressing on the standing knee joint, and be careful to keep the hips level. Focus on an object (preferably not someone else in your yoga class or yourself in the mirror but an inanimate object that won't move and make you lose your balance!) and bring the palms together into prayer pose, or the Namaste mudra. You can also lift your arms above the head into a diamond shape, or from the diamond open the arms outward like branches of a tree. RR. Again, your balance will be tested, but once you attain the position you will find a great sense of focus mentally and physically. For a more challenging version of Tree, which for some people is easier to balance, bend the knee of the free leg and bring the foot to the hipbone of the standing leg. This is almost like a Standing Half Lotus position. Try to keep the toes open in lotus flower position as the foot presses isometrically against the upper leg/hip bone.

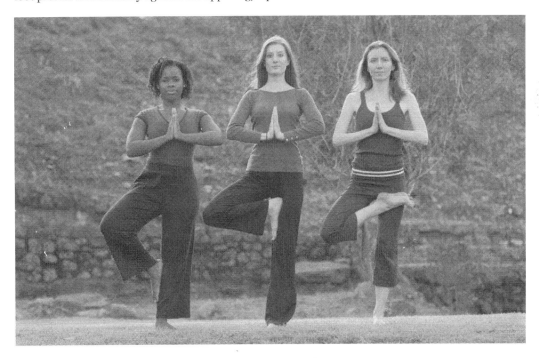

Like in Schubert's "Der Lindenbaum" (Linden Tree): There you would have found peace!

CHAPTER 3

## BRIDGE

This inversion helps with stacking the spine as you roll up and down through the vertebrae. Rolling through the vertebrae has a calming effect which can ameliorate performance anxiety.

Lying on your back with your knees bent and feet close to the buttocks, slowly raise the hips as you lift your lower, middle and then upper back off the floor. To release, slowly lower the spine vertebra by vertebra. Rolling through the vertebrae gently massages them while heightening your awareness of the individual components that make up the spinal column. You can also try Bridge with your hands clasped underneath you: bring the shoulder blades closer together and roll your shoulders outwards so they are bearing some weight and lift the sternum, providing reinforcement of a lifted and expansive chest. It is very important to keep the noble chest posture so that no pressure is placed on the neck and larynx.

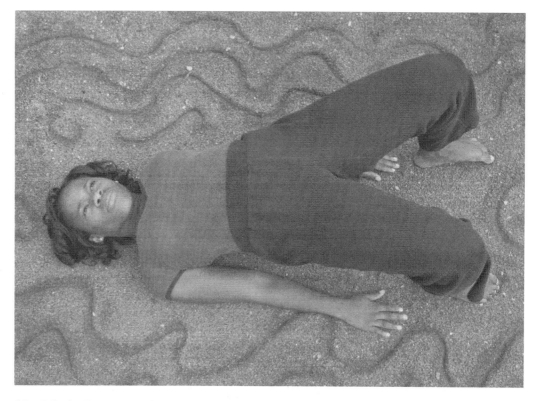

"Like a Bridge Over Troubled Water." –Simon and Garfunkel

62

# Forward Bends

Besides stretching the legs, these poses soothe the spine, shoulders, and spirit when you surrender to their challenges. By confronting your body's struggle with these poses, your psyche learns not to run from physical resistance, just as you don't want your mind to flee when there is the mental/emotional battle of stage fright. As you explore forward bends, try not to round the spine but keep it long, imagining a flat, table-top back. Remember to hold each stretch for at least thirty seconds and use your breath to go deeper into the stretch. After a long, slow inhalation, exhale as you try to stretch a bit further. Remember that pain is a sign that you are pushing your body too far, so never stretch to the point of pain. In yoga, seated forward bends are usually done with flexed feet.

## HEAD-TO-KNEE POSE

Sit in Staff pose. Bend the left knee, bringing the left foot to your right inner thigh. Keeping the right leg straight, reach out over the extended leg. It is almost like doing Tree in a seated position. RR. This is a good way to ease into the effort of forward bends. Your body will resist but will release if you approach your practice with patience and apply the use of your breath.

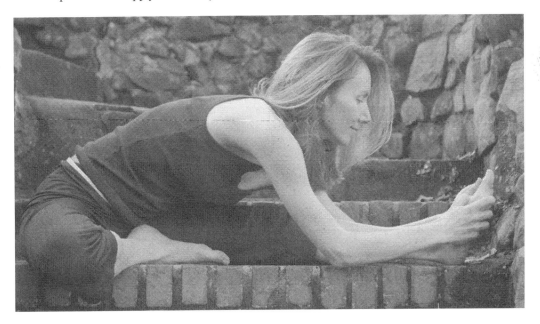

"Head, shoulders, knees and toes." —Children's bus song

## SEATED FORWARD BEND

Sit in Staff pose. Bend forward stretching towards the feet. Try not to round the spine but keep it long (think of bringing your lower belly to your thighs), and bring the shoulders down away from the ears. This will be more challenging than head-to-knee pose, but you will stretch the back of the legs (the hamstrings) even more and this will help you with strength and length in standing. Feel free to use a yoga strap if you need. Wrap the strap around the soles of your flexed feet and use it to pull gently forward towards the feet.

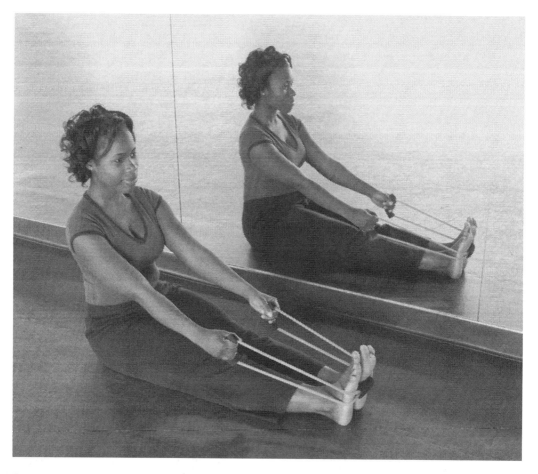

"Learning How to Bend." —country singer Gary Allan

# STANDING FORWARD BEND

From Mountain pose, reach the arms up and overhead into Tall Mountain. With a flat back, gently bend forward from the hips and reach the torso towards the knees. The hands reach towards the toes or touch the ground. Or you can clasp your elbows for a "rag doll" position, which can help relieve shoulder and neck tension. As with Seated forward bend, try to roll the shoulders back away from the ears. If you have a back injury, be careful to try this pose first with bent knees. This stretch adds so much suppleness to the spine because gravity can help you with the lengthening and strengthening of the back muscles. Also, the weight of the head helps stretch the back of the neck. After doing this intense hamstring stretch, roll up to standing and feel like you are stacking your vertebrae on long energized legs. Imagine a string (or the shakti serpent) extending from your heel up your Achilles tendon into the hamstring and all the way up through the spine.

Here are two more advanced variations of the asana: try the pose with the back of your legs near a wall, using its verticality to deepen the stretch; or try the pose with your back near a wall and walk gingerly as close to the wall as you can so that your back and legs are almost parallel with the wall.

These intense variations are not for beginners, but they can provide a deep, rewarding release in the often stubborn hamstrings.

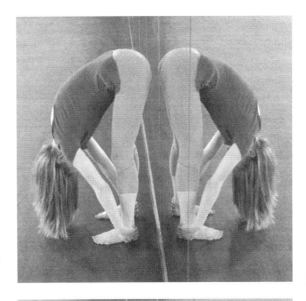

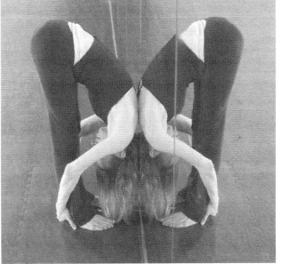

"How can I go forward when I don't know which way I'm facing?"
–John Lennon

# WIDE-LEGGED STANDING FORWARD BEND (or STRADDLE)

From Mountain pose, open the legs into a wide stance. Stretch the back straight and long as you reach downwards, clasping your arms at your elbows and letting yourself hang over. For a more advanced stretch, widen your stance and gently rest your head on the floor or on a block. This pose uses gravity to lengthen and take pressure off the spine. Try to replicate this feeling when you are standing upright. Wide-legged standing forward bend can also help concentration by stimulating blood flow to the brain. It is also thought to help relieve headaches and mild depression.

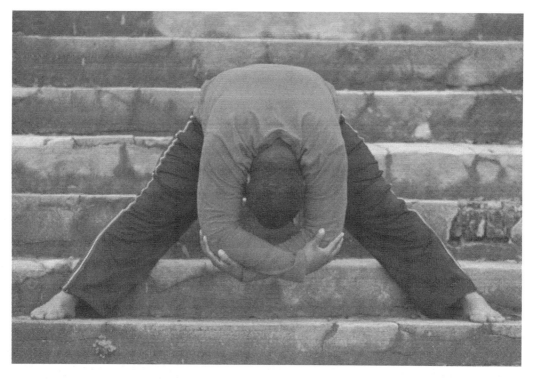

"Bend and Not Break." –Dashboard Confessional

## WIDE OR OPEN ANGLE SEATED
## FORWARD BEND

From Staff pose open the legs into a V. Without rounding the spine
(think of bringing your lower belly to the floor), reach the hands
towards the feet and stretch the torso over the floor in front of you.
Trying to keep your arms long, rest your hands where you can on your
knees, shins, toes or on the floor in front of you. The more flexible and/
or advanced practitioner may want to rest the chest or forehead on the
floor or open the legs wider in a center split. As you do this version of
forward bends, be aware of the length of all four limbs and try to keep
them all fully extended. Then try to bring this sense of extension and
elongation to your arms and legs when in your regular standing posture. Long legs, long arms, and a long spine will create a wonderful
stance onstage and will underpin the solidity of your structural alignment for singing.

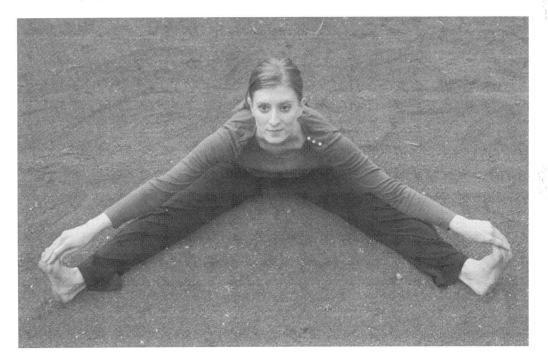

Madonna opens her "Hung Up" video by stretching into Wide-legged forward bend.

# Rib-opening Asanas

As you approach these asanas, focus on creating space between the ribs by expanding the intercostals (the muscles in between the ribs) and thus increasing the circumference of the rib cage. Good singing alignment involves a high, noble chest and sternum. It is important to keep the rib cage elevated and the ribs expanded so that the lungs are unimpeded and thus free to inflate fully. Singing demands the breath control to sustain the prolonged exhalation of long sung phrases, and this breath control is reliant on maintaining the expansion of the lungs. Besides helping with posture and breathing, having an open/wide chest is inviting to the audience as you are showing the audience everything that you are, not hiding behind a closed position with the shoulders rolled forward and the chest collapsed. Your voice teacher may even espouse rib breathing. Regardless of your approach, expanded and unimpeded ribs are beneficial to breathing and necessary for good breathing for singing. If, like most of us, you weren't granted a barrel chest at birth, then imagine you have the cavernous rib cage of legendary Swedish tenor Jussi Björling, or the more contemporary Italian opera star Salvatore Licitra, or even Johnny Cash.

# GATE AND REVERSE GATE

Open the gate to open ribs, and open the door to singing longer phrases without rib collapse.

From Hero, rise up onto the knees. Extend the right leg directly to the side, opening the right hip but keeping the sole of the right foot on the floor. Lift the arms overhead and extend the upper body over the right leg, resting the right arm on the right leg and stretching the left arm over the right leg. You should feel a stretch in your left side, but be careful to keep the right side as long as you can and not crunched. Keep the top arm from crossing in front of the chest and collapsing the rib cage. For Reverse Gate (which is also a variation on Side Plank) lift the torso and bring the arms overhead. Place the left hand on the floor leaning the torso the other direction away from the extended right leg. Reach the right arm to the left stretching the other side of the rib cage. Release the arms overhead and sit back into Hero. RR. Imagine your rib cage is like an opening gate, or like a rainbow extending its colorful arc in a sweeping curve. Gate is perhaps the most effective prescription for singers who struggle with a collapsed rib cage.

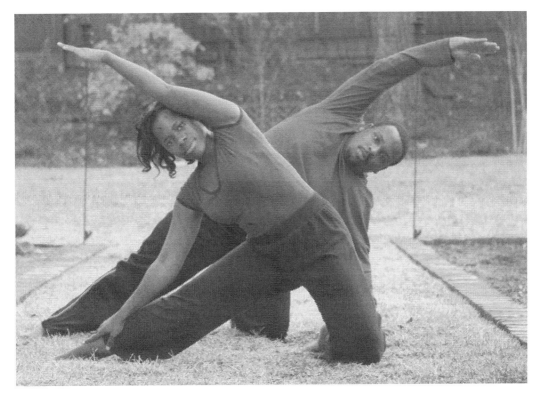

"Open the Gate." —No Doubt

## SIDE PLANK

Rib expansion, shoulder strength, and balance all-in-one: a triptych of benefits for triple-threat performers!

Prepare for Reverse Gate (right leg extended) making sure the left hand is directly beneath the left shoulder. Once the left arm is extended and you have your balance, move the left leg so that the left foot is stacked beneath the right. RR. You should feel like you are pushing powerfully away from the ground to lift and open the chest. This pose also has the spinal alignment benefits of regular or reverse plank.

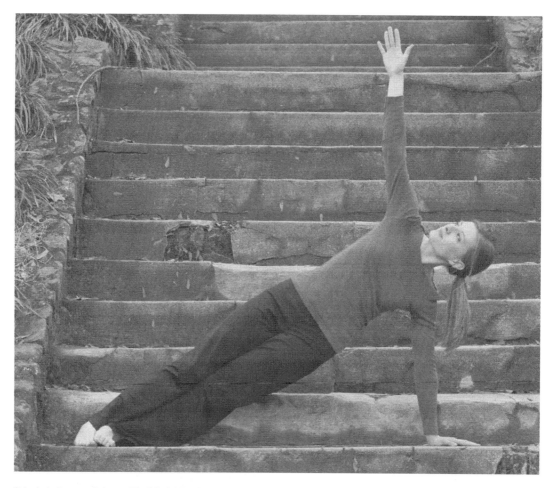

Side plank always reminds me of the Jets dancing through the streets in *West Side Story*.

# TRIANGLE

A great standing stretch for the rib cage, creating the expansion necessary for good breath control.

Standing in Mountain, turn out the right foot (and hip) perpendicular to the left foot. Then move the right foot 3-4 feet away from the left foot and lift the arms to the sides. Keeping the legs straight and the hips facing to the side, bend from the hip joint and lower the upper body over the right leg. Rest the right hand on the calf, on a block or on the floor (or on a stair-step, as in the photograph). Look up at the ceiling (or to the sky if you have the pleasure of practicing yoga outdoors). Focus on keeping the rib cage wide and expanded, and make sure the sternum doesn't collapse. To come out of Triangle, look down at the foot and gently lift the upper body. RR. Triangle lets you focus on one half of the rib cage at a time by making you aware of the ribs twisting and reaching up to the ceiling. As with rib-cage isolations in dance, focusing on one body part improves your awareness of it and your ability to isolate and work on very specific muscles. For an even more intense rib spreading experience, bring the upper arm around behind the back, bend at the elbow and reach around (to try) to find the top of the front thigh. Known as "binding," this technique provides a sensation of length and width at the waist which is especially helpful for more petite singers of slender girth who often have trouble maintaining the expansion necessary for good breath support.

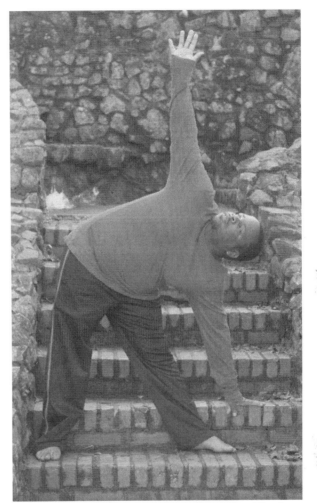

Triangle pose evokes the Masonic Pyramid and triadic symbolism of Mozart's *Die Zauberflöte*.

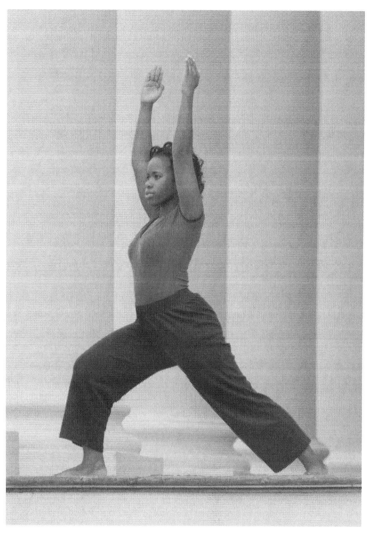

"I am the Warrior." –Patty Smyth

## WARRIOR 1

Stretches and strengthens the chest, neck, and shoulders, all prime areas of tension for singers.

From Mountain, step into a forward lunge with the right foot, leaving the left heel down. (Some schools of yoga prefer to lift the back heel so you can lunge more deeply in Warrior I or a Crescent Lunge.) With the hips facing forward and the front knee directly over the front toe, bend the right knee into a right angle. Lifting the rib cage away from the pelvis, extend the arms straight overhead. RR. Focus on lifting the sternum and keeping the shoulders rolled down and back, just like you will want in your stance for singing.

# WARRIOR 2

Also known as Proud Warrior.

From Mountain, step into a forward lunge with the right foot. Keeping the left/back heel down turn the hips open to the left as you lift the arms parallel to the ground. Make sure the torso does not lean over the front leg and focus on extending the arms away from each other in one long horizontal line. RR. This empowering pose for singers lifts and separates the pectoral muscles, providing a wide, barrel-chested feeling. Warrior 2 is often approached from Warrior 1. To transition from Warrior 1 to 2, open the hips and arms to the side and deepen the bend in the front knee while you gaze over the fingertips of your front hand.

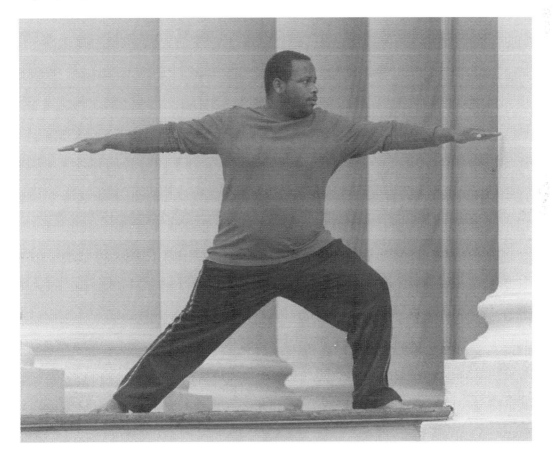

Think of the proud warrior Radames in Giuseppe Verdi's (or Elton John's) *Aïda*.

## SIDE ANGLE POSE

Lengthen from (finger) tip to (toe) tip, and sing with a longer-feeling torso.

From Warrior 2, lower the front (left in the photo) hand to the ground behind the front (left) foot or to the thigh or a yoga block. Then stretch the right arm up and over to form a straight line all the way from the right heel to the right hand fingertips. RR. Be sure not to round or collapse the torso forward. Side Angle pose combines the rib-opening benefits of Triangle and Gate with the spinal alignment awareness of Side Plank.

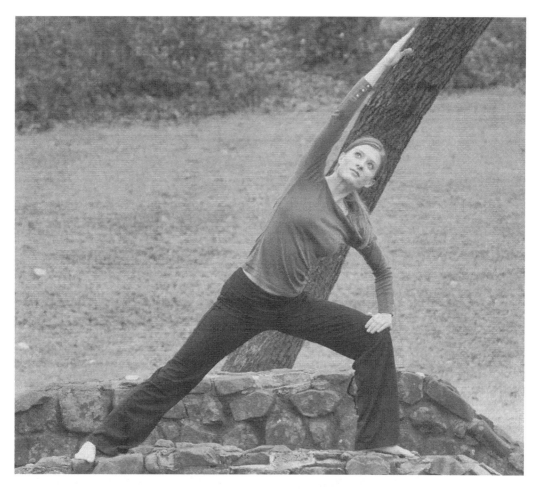

Find the critical Angle of Repose to experimental band Sleepytime Gorilla Museum's "Angle of Repose."

# REVOLVED SIDE ANGLE

Adds a spinal twist to rotate the rib stretch, lengthening the trunk while calming singers' nerves through the spinal rotation.

From Side Angle (right foot forward), turn the torso to the right. Place the left hand on the outside of the right foot and extend the right arm straight up as you gaze upwards. RR. By revolving or rotating the side angle, you get to stretch the other side. This allows you to focus on one side of the rib cage at a time, expanding and stretching each in turn. Perform Side Angle and Revolved Side Angle on both sides, and you have built a strong foundation for ample rib expansion.

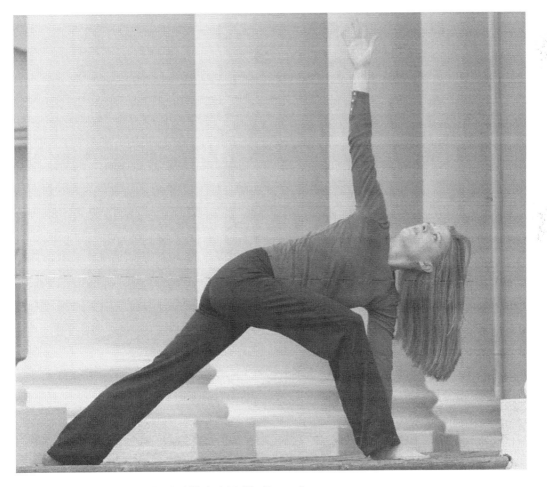

Coldplay singer Chris Martin has done Revolved Side Angle into Wheel in concert.

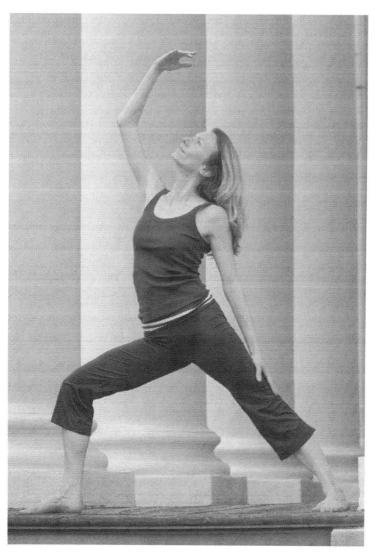

Reverse Warrior is my favorite "Diva Warrior" pose.

# REVERSE WARRIOR

Spread and stretch the intercostals for an invigorated stage stance.

From Warrior 2, keep the back arm extended backwards but lower it to the back leg as you lift the front arm overhead and gently arch upwards and backwards. Focus on the intense expansion of the rib cage. Reverse Warrior adds the rib-intensity of Gate pose and pectoral expansion of Proud Warrior to a lifted sternum and frontal spinal stretch. Combining the empowerment of Warrior with the strengthening stretch of a backbend, Reverse Warrior is another one of my favorite asanas thanks to its energizing and focusing properties. Reverse Warrior always makes me think of the Degas painting "Singer with a Glove" and was the inspiration for the cover of this book.

# COW FACE

Opens the chest and stretches the shoulders and triceps.

Sitting with the legs crossed and the knees stacked on each other (or in Hero or Lotus), reach the left arm behind you, placing the left hand between the shoulders blades with the palm facing away from the body. Lift the right arm straight up and then bend at the elbow. Reach the hands toward each other and if possible, clasp the hands together. You can also use a yoga strap between the hands if the hands cannot touch. Be sure not to collapse the chest or jut the neck forward. RR. Besides helping to lift and expand the chest, Cow face helps relieve stress on the shoulders, which can become rigid trying to maintain proper rib and sternum elevation. A side benefit of mastering Cow face is the ability to put sun block on any part of your own back! I suppose this could also come in handy for applying your own body makeup if you were playing Salome or Lakmé. Or if you are a perennially shirtless divo like buff baritone Nathan Gunn or my colleague Chuck Schneider who, instead of Shoeless Joe from Hannibal, MO, was shirtless Hal from KS for almost all of Act I of Libby Larsen's opera *Picnic*.

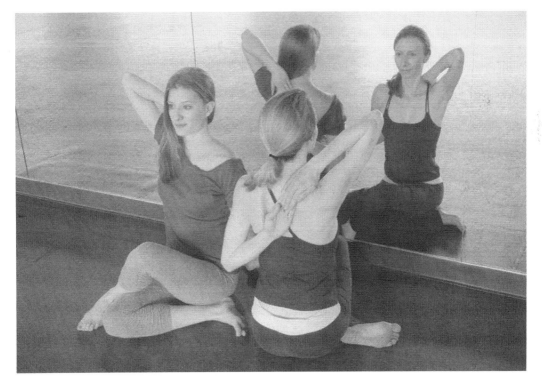

Be like Jack's cow in Stephen Sondheim's *Into the Woods*.

## FISH

Wonderful for helping to develop the singer's noble posture of a high sternum.

From Corpse, bring your elbows into the rib cage. Keeping the hips on the floor, arch backwards and roll gently onto the crown of the head. Be sure to keep weight on your elbows and not the neck. You don't want to put any pressure on the precious larynx! Fish is often done with the feet in Diamond/Goddess pose, with the soles of the feet together as if you were doing Bound Angle pose supine (as in the photograph). Typically the counter pose to Shoulder stand, it can also be done with the legs extended as in Corpse pose. In addition to opening the shoulders, ribs, and chest, Fish provides a nice, gentle stretch for the front of the neck.

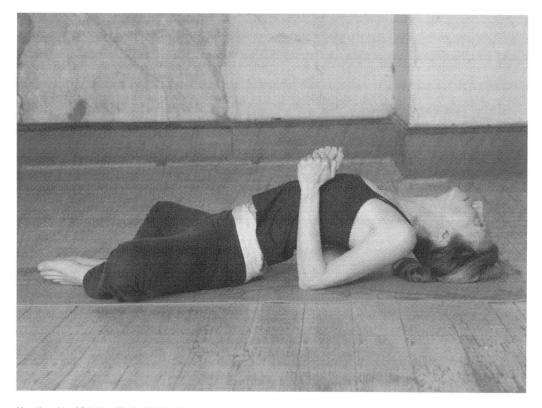

More thoughts of Schubert: "Die Forelle" (The Trout).

## COBRA

Akin to a Mini Up Dog, but with more focus on the chest and upper back than the spine.

Lie on your belly and place the palms of your hands on the floor beneath the shoulders. Keeping the elbows bent and close into the rib cage, lift the forearms, head, neck, and upper back off the floor. (If you leave the forearms on the floor, then it is Sphinx Pose, as in the photograph. The hips remain on the floor, otherwise it becomes Up Dog.) Cobra forces you to focus on rolling the shoulders back in their proper alignment. For an additional challenge, lift the hands to fully engage the muscles of your upper back. Strengthening these upper back muscles keeps them in balance with the shoulders and will help you maintain your good standing posture.

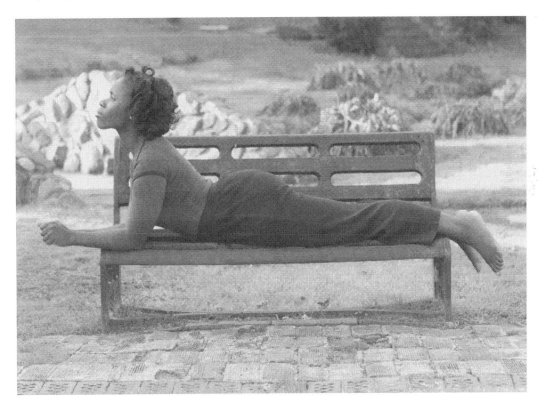

A sinewy snake like in the musical *The Apple Tree* or Lee Hoiby's song "The Serpent."

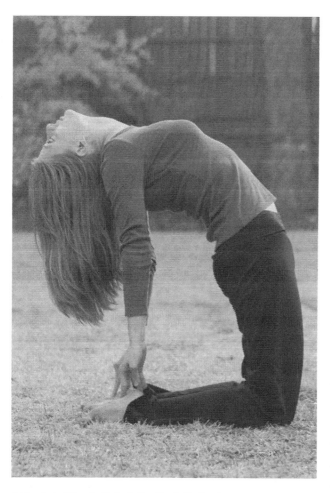

Kristian Bush of Sugarland is fond of backbends like Camel.

## CAMEL

A kneeling form of Bow pose and preparation for Wheel (a full back-bend as in gymnastics, and one of Madonna's favorite poses), Camel helps prevent slumped posture in singers. To create the look of a dromedary hump, ironically the pose arches the back into a convex rather than concave curvature.

From Hero, rise up onto the knees. Gently arch backwards and place the palms on the lower back, helping to expand and stretch the arch without compressing the spine. As you keep the sternum lifted, reach the right hand back to rest on the sole or heel of the right foot (Half Camel). For Full Camel, reach the left hand back to the left foot. Release carefully, being sure to use core abdominal strength to lift out of the arch. After this intense backward stretch, rest in Child's pose. Like other back-bends, Camel combats the tendency to slouch or round the spine and is a wonderful antidote for those with collapsed sternums and/or ribs. Still, in Camel you should feel as if you are arching yet lifting upwards instead of bending backwards in order to keep the expansion of the intercostals and maximize this pose's rib-spreading effect. To make the pose easier, curl the toes under, which brings the heels closer to the hands in the backward arch. For the more challenging version of Camel, keep the tops of the feet flat on the floor.

# (Especially) Singer-friendly Asanas

## LION POSE

A wonderful stretch and release for singers with jaw and/or tongue tension.

(Esteemed voice teacher Cynthia Hoffmann, on faculty at Juilliard and the Manhattan School of Music, reportedly uses Lion as a body warm-up in a typical lesson.)

Start in Hero pose, then kneel. With Bob Fosse jazz hands or *Bring It On* spirit fingers, place the palms of your hands on your knees. Inhale and look up between your eyebrows, at what is sometimes called the "third eye." As you begin to exhale on an [h ]*d*, stick out your tongue and stretch it towards your chin. Lion is an ideal asana to do before beginning to vocalize since it can help release the tongue and open the throat. Be careful not to stretch the tongue too forcefully. Remember that the tongue is attached to the larynx (the irreplaceable jewels or, as one of my voice teachers called it, the money!) so try to extend the tongue without pressing it. This asana is helpful for singers who tend to pull the tongue back or who struggle with a tight, tremulous tongue while singing. Spreading the fingers is supposed to encourage the tongue to spread and stay wide instead of constricting and shaking. Plus, Lion creates awareness of *gola aperta* (open throat) as air moves through the vocal tract during the Lion's Roar.

---

*d* Text in [brackets] implies IPA, the International Phonetic Alphabet.

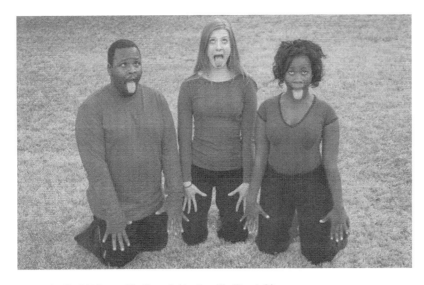

Be *The Lion King's* Mufasa, not the Cowardly Lion from *The Wizard of Oz*.

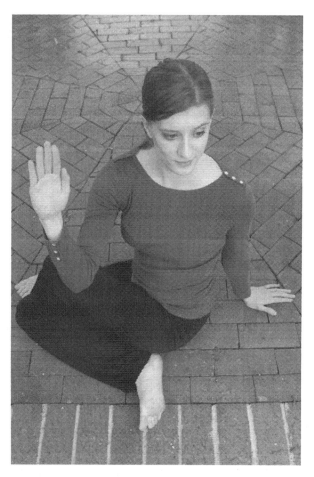

Stretch through Elgar's *Sea Pictures* or the *Sea Symphony* by Vaughan Williams.

# SPINAL TWISTS

Like a good massage therapy session, these poses calm the mind and nervous system, help to balance energy, and relieve head and neck tension. Spinal twists are also associated with awakening Kundalini energy. Think of your body pulling in two different directions to stretch, unwind, and uncoil the spinal column. Be sure to breathe as you perform these asanas, exhaling into the twist. These twists seem to minimize some people's need for chiropractic adjustments. Since they move and massage the digestive organs, it is not recommended to do these twists on a full stomach, but they make a wonderful addition to a pre-performance preparation ritual. Instead of "Twist and Shout," Twist and Sing!

## HALF LORD OF THE FISHES

From Half Lotus with right leg on top, lift the right leg and place the right foot on the floor next to the left outer thigh. Be sure to keep the right hip on the floor. Place the left elbow on the outside of the right knee and twist the torso to the right as you rest the right hand on the floor behind you. Be sure to keep the shoulders level. Your gaze should follow the direction of the twist. RR. Half Lord of the Fishes helps to energize the spine and thus discourages slouching. For an apropos and amusing image, imagine salmon swimming upstream through your spine as you twist.

# LYING SPINAL TWIST

From Corpse, hug the right knee while keeping the left leg extended. Place the left hand on the outside of the right knee and bring the knee to the left side, twisting the torso to the left and extending the right arm along the floor to your right. Look towards your right hand. The right knee can touch the ground if possible, but be sure to keep your right shoulder on the floor. RR. This spine soothing twist is especially helpful in releasing the lower back before Corpse pose. From an overhead view, this pose is reminiscent of a Busby Berkeley showgirl pose.

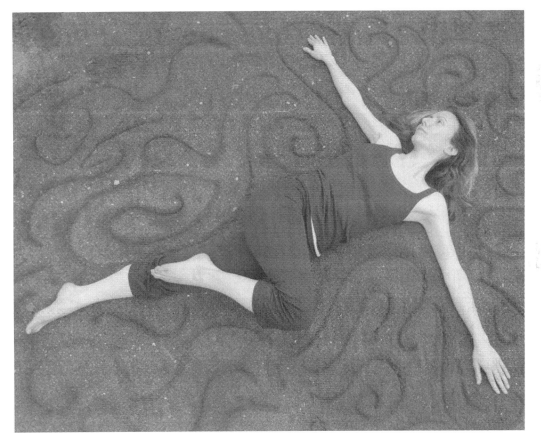

"Lie Down in the Light."– folk singer Bonnie 'Prince' Billy

## CHILD'S POSE WITH THREAD THE NEEDLE

From Hero, start to reach the left arm forward into Child's pose as you slide the right arm (palm up) beneath it to the left at a ninety degree angle. The head rests on the floor on the right cheek. RR. In addition to its spinal twist, this pose provides a greatly restorative shoulder stretch. If the stretch is too intense, you could place a block or blanket under the shoulders.

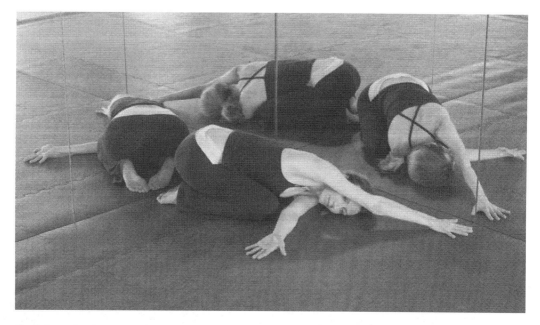

"Here's the needle and thread to mend your broken heart." –Lit

## CHAIR PRAYER TWIST

From Mountain lift the arms straight overhead as you bend the knees
to sit into Chair pose. Keeping the knees together and hips forward,
place the palms of the hands together into Prayer and turn the upper
body to the right. Place the left elbow on the outside of the right knee
and keep turning the torso as you look up at the ceiling. RR. This
asana unites the centering of a balancing pose with the calming effect
of the spinal twist. Plus the mudra or hand position has other harmonizing properties (as will be discussed in Chapter Four). Prayer Twist
befits the supplications of Puccini's *Suor Angelica* and the beleaguered
Blanche in Poulenc's *Dialogues of the Carmelites*, two operatic roles
requiring great dramatic and vocal focus and fortitude.

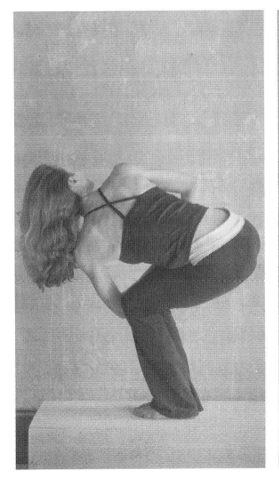
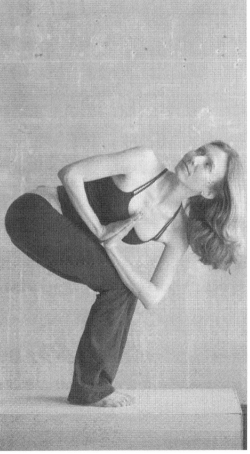

"Say a Prayer for Me Tonight." –Lerner and Loewe's *Gigi*

## LUNGE or EQUESTRIAN PRAYER TWIST

From Mountain, lunge the right foot forward lifting the left heel (Equestrian Pose). Keeping the hips forward place the palms of the hands together into Prayer and twist the upper body to the right. Place the left elbow on the outside of the right knee and keep turning the torso as you look up at the ceiling. RR. Equestrian Prayer twist is good for those who find Chair Prayer Twist too winding or tortuous. If are having trouble balancing or need to lessen the intensity of the pose, let the back knee rest on the floor. As its name indicates, this asana is great just before jumping on a horse, or on Billy Bigelow's *Carousel*.

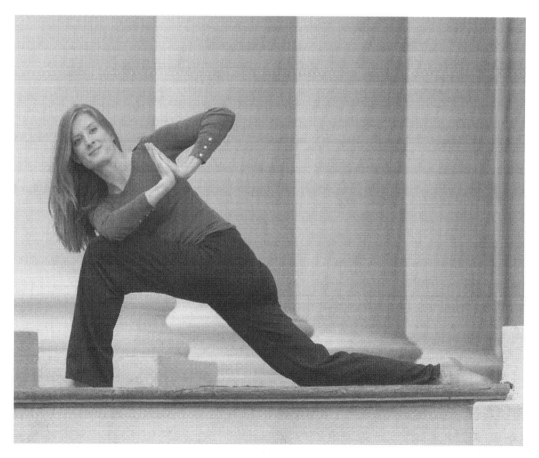

"Give a Man a Horse He Can Ride." –Geoffrey O'Hara

# REVOLVED TRIANGLE

From Mountain move the right foot 3-4 feet to the front aligning the right and left heels. Both feet are in parallel and the hips should stay facing front even as the triangle revolves. Raise the arms to the side parallel to the floor and bend over at the waist with a flat back. Make sure the hips are facing forward as you turn the upper body to the right. Place the left hand on the calf, on a block, or on the floor (or on a stair-step) as your reach the right hand to the ceiling and gaze up at it. RR. Revolved Triangle helps to open the chest and improve balance. It massages the lower back, which should help alignment of the spine, and is even thought to help relieve the symptoms of mild asthma.

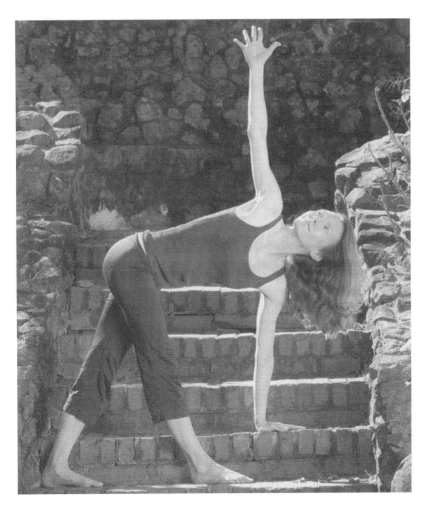

"Turn, turn, turn." –Pete Seeger

## SHOULDER STAND/PLOW

A challenging but rewarding inversion which increases calmness and concentration. Besides stretching the neck and shoulders, it also helps alleviate stress and sinusitis, two common plagues for singers.

From L pose, place the palms on the back of the legs. Gently walk the hands down your body to your back as you lift the legs toward the ceiling. Keep the elbows bent as you support yourself on your shoulders. Try to get as straight up and down as possible (as high onto your shoulders as possible). For an additional spinal stretch, as Jon Cryer's character Ducky says in *Pretty in Pink*, "let's plow." For Plow pose, lower the legs behind the head until your toes touch the floor (or a block or a chair behind you). Keep the legs straight, or bend the knees and draw them into the ears. (To release, gently walk the hands down the spine and lower your spine back to the floor.) Shoulder stand can help singers in developing mental focus as well as enhancing their perception of spinal alignment. The inversion of Shoulder stand and Plow helps calm the mind and may even help reduce sinusitis. It is traditional to do Fish pose after Shoulder stand since it acts as an effective counter pose.

IMPORTANT NOTE: *DO NOT turn or twist the neck while in Shoulder stand or Plow. Avoid these poses if you have had a neck injury and stick to L pose for the benefits of an inverted asana.*

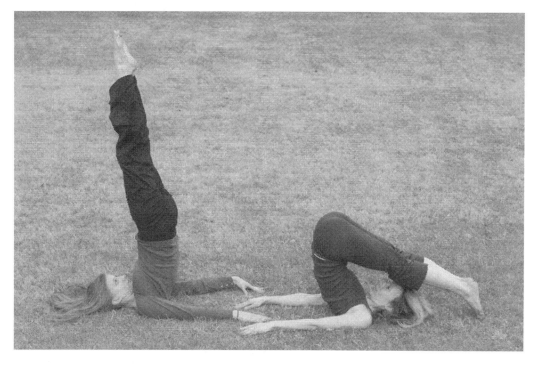

Shoulder stand (left); Plow (right), which Rihanna does in her "Rude Boy" video.

# Vinyasas

Hold each pose for a count of 2 to 10 depending on the speed and intensity you want for your flow: the faster the flow then the greater the intensity, the slower the flow the more time you have to focus on form. Be sure to use props as necessary to maximize your form in the asanas. Also, focus on maintaining a clearly defined breath cycle of steady inhalation and exhalation. Never "hold" your breath as your "hold" a pose.

## 1. spine stretching

The Spine Stretcher vinyasas are a combination of forward and backward bends designed to elongate the spine and make it supple and strong. The benefits of these flows are improved spinal alignment and a strong, well-supported back for energy and length in your spine and thus your stance onstage.

### SPINE STRETCHER 1
### (Standing and Balancing)

- Mountain.
- Tree.
- Tall Mountain.
- Warrior Three.
- Tall Mountain.
- Swan dive into Standing forward bend.
- Hop into Plank.
- Lower body to the ground then lift the chest into Up Dog.
- Lift the hips into Down Dog.
- Hop the feet together for Standing forward bend.
- Lift and return to Mountain.

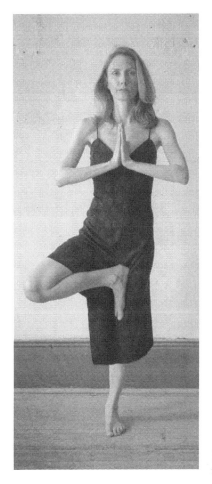

Tree.

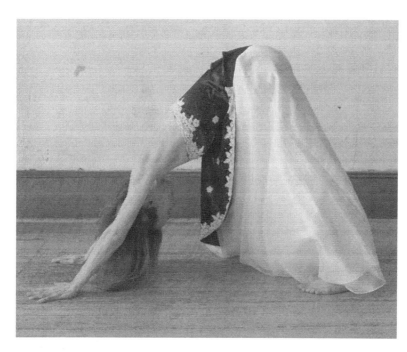

Down Dog.

## SPINE STRETCHER 2 (Upward and Backward Bends)

• Hero.

• Cow.

• Cat.

• Cow.

• Cat.

• Child's pose.

• Locust.

• Bow.

• Up Dog.

• Down Dog.

• Hop the feet open into Wide-Legged Standing Forward Bend.

• Hop the feet together and roll the spine up into Mountain.

## SPINE STRETCHER 3
### (Seated and Forward Bends)

- Staff.
- Head to knee pose (right side).
- Staff.
- Seated forward bend.
- Head to knee pose (left side).
- Staff.
- Reverse plank.
- Seated forward bend.
- Roll back into Corpse.
- Bend the knees and bring the feet into the buttocks to lift into Bridge. Gently lower. Repeat Bridge or lift into a full backbend (Wheel pose).

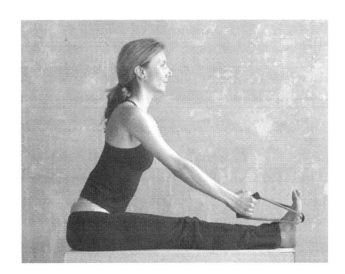

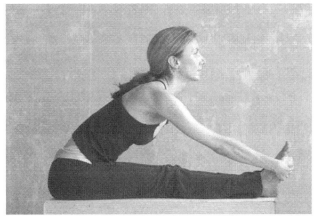

Seated Forward Bend (with and without yoga strap).

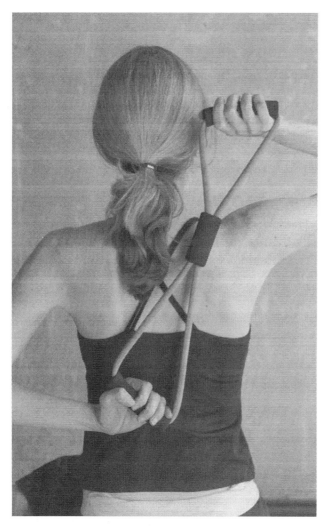

Cow face pose (with yoga strap).

# 2. rib spreading

For the Rib spreading vinyasas, expand and open the rib cage by concentrating on lifting the sternum and engaging the intercostals. These asana sequences assist more efficient breathing since they reinforce the sensation of a wide rib cage with room for unimpeded lung expansion and the increased ability to sing lengthy Mozartean melismas, long, sustained Jerome Kern melodies, or extended gospel licks.

## RIB SPREADER 1 (Seated and Kneeling)

- Hero.
- Cow face.
- Lion.
- Gate and Reverse Gate.
- Camel.
- Child's pose.
- Side plank and Thread the Needle with Child (both sides).
- Hero.

## RIB SPREADER 2
## (Standing: Warrior Series)

• Mountain.

• Swan dive into Standing forward bend.

• Hop into Plank, then lower to prone.

• Lift into Up Dog, then Down Dog.

• Bring the right foot forward to step into Warrior 1.

• Turn the left hip open into Warrior 2, then lower the front arm to Triangle
  Pose. (or Side Angle Pose).

• Lift into Reverse Warrior.

• Step into Warrior 3.

• Step into Mountain.

• RR.

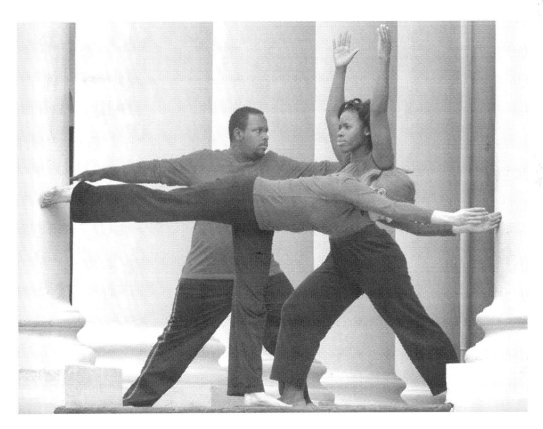

Warrior Series.

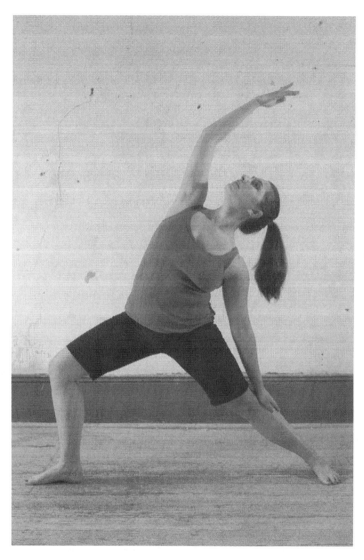

Reverse Warrior.

## RIB SPREADER 3 (Revolving Rib Sun Salutation)

• Mountain.
• Swan dive into Standing forward bend. Hop into Plank, then lower to prone.
• Lift into Up Dog, then Down Dog.
• Bring the right foot forward and rotate the torso to the right for Revolved Triangle.
• Bend the right knee, lower the left knee into a lunge (Equestrian pose) and bring the palms together for Lunge Prayer Twist.
• Release to center.
• Side Angle Pose.
• Reverse Warrior.
• Revolved Side Angle.
• Chair prayer twist.
• Chair.
• Mountain.
• RR.

## ADVANCED SPINE STRETCHER AND RIB SPREADER
### (Sun Salutation with Shoulder Stand)

• Mountain.

• Chair with prayer twist.

• Tall Mountain.

• Swan dive into Standing forward bend.

• Hop into Plank.

• Lift to Side Plank on each side.

• Return to Plank and lower to prone.

• Lift into Cobra, then Up Dog and Down Dog.

• Hop feet open into Standing forward bend.

• Bend knees to hop into Staff.

• Lift into Reverse Plank.

• Lower and lie back into Corpse.

• Lift legs into L pose.

• Lift into Shoulder stand and/or Plow (if desired).

• Roll down into Corpse.

• Fish.

• Corpse.

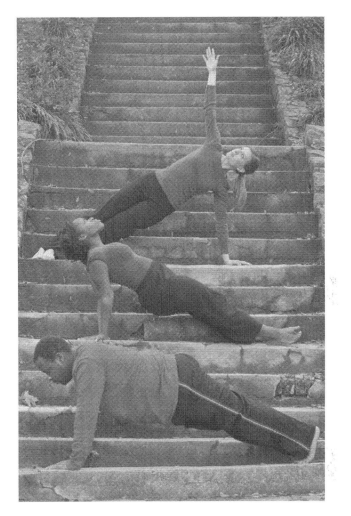

Plank Series.

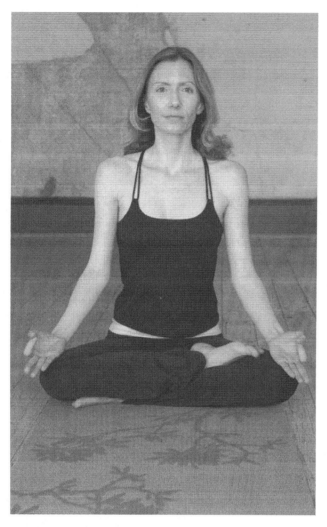

Half Lotus.

# 3. spine soothing

These Spine soothers massage the spine, calm the nerves, and help focus the mind. They are particularly helpful before a performance to help relieve stress and anxiety while heightening focus and concentration.

## SPINE SOOTHER 1 (Useful right before meditation in Half or Full Lotus pose)

- Start in Bound Angle.
- Cross the right leg over for Half Lord of the Fishes.
- Lift the right leg in your arms (Rock the baby), setting it on the left the leg into Half Lotus or into Full Lotus if you desire.
- RR.

## SPINE SOOTHER 2
### (Useful right before meditation in Corpse pose)

• Start in Corpse.
• Hug the right knee and roll the body over to the left for Lying Spinal Twist.
• Return to center and repeat with the left leg.
• Hug both knees and gently roll them in circles massaging the spine.
• Extend the legs into Corpse.

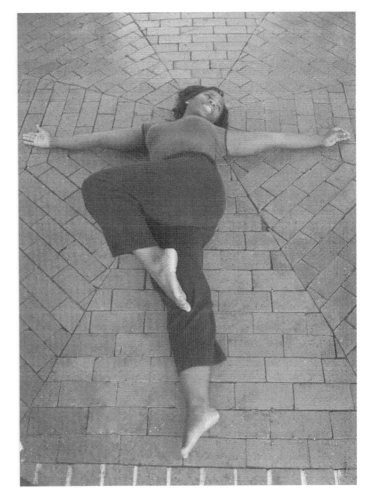

Lying Spinal Twist.

## ADVANCED SPINE SOOTHER
### (Spinal twists with Shoulder Stand)

- Start in Staff.
- Open the legs and stretch into Open or Wide Angle Seated Forward Bend.
- Return to Staff and roll back into Corpse.
- Hug the right knee and roll the body over to the left for Lying Spinal Twist.
- Return to center and repeat with the left leg.
- Hug both knees and gently roll them in circles massaging the spine.
- Bridge.
- Lift the legs into L pose or Shoulder stand and Plow.
- Release and roll down.
- Fish.
- Corpse.

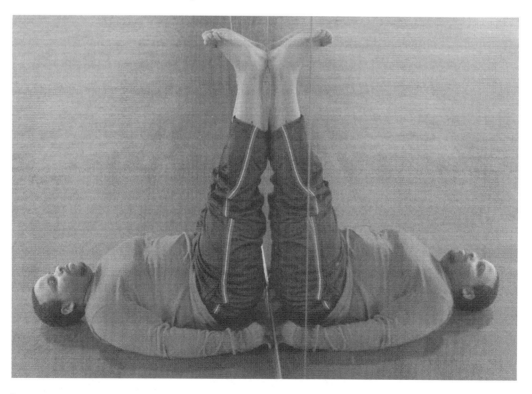

L pose.

# BACKSTAGE VINYASA

**(omit any asanas which might jeopardize your costume or concert attire!)**

This standing vinyasa is suitable for doing backstage before making your entrance for an opera, musical, or concert.

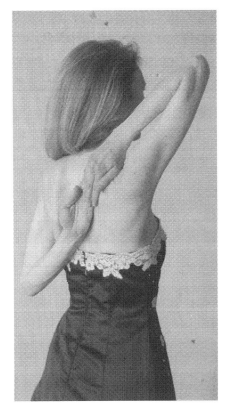

Cow Face.

• Remove your shoes and start in Mountain pose.

• Lift arms into a standing version of Gate pose.

• RR.

• Stretch the shoulders by doing the arm stretch of Cow Face while standing.

• If there is enough room backstage, open your stance to do Warrior 2 (Proud Warrior), Triangle or Side Angle pose, Down Dog, and standing forward bend.

• Roll up slowly, stacking the vertebrae.

• Try Tree, with the foot at the calf instead of the thigh if necessary.

• RR.

• End with Lion pose and some Ujjayi breathing.

• Either sitting on a chair or in Lotus, try some meditation to combat any performance anxiety/stage fright.

• Make your entrance and sing with calm confidence!

Practice these asanas alone and/or in the recommended vinyasas to see improvement in the quality and strength of your postural alignment. You will feel taller with a longer, stronger spine, a wider rib cage, and a free yet centered spirit.

# 4

## Meditation: Mantras and Mudras

*"Yoga is the method by which the restless mind is calmed and the energy directed into constructive channels."*

—B.K.S. Iyengar

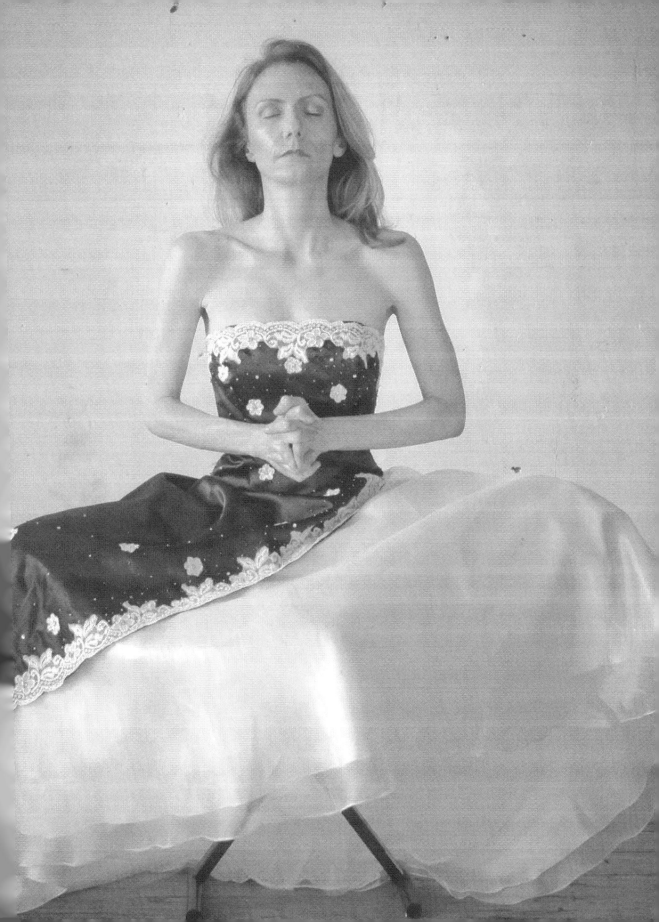

*"Vanessa Williams is <u>amazing</u>. She brought her yoga instructor to do yoga between shows. She's not a crazy diva. She's so zen."*

—**Stephen DeRosa**, *Vanessa's co-star in the Broadway revival of the musical "Into the Woods"*

Scientific study has revealed meditation to be a powerful and potent stress reliever. Not surprisingly, meditation can provide a compelling method for combating and coping with performance anxiety. The practice of meditation provides coping skills to deal with the common fight or flight mechanism of stage fright, preventing adverse physical reactions such as an elevated heart rate and shallow breathing. Moreover, as mentioned before, meditation can help singers to fight detrimental psychological reactions as well, helping to eliminate negative and unnecessary thoughts that might hinder their ability to remember text or perform at their optimal level.

So what is meditation? It is most commonly defined as the act of thinking deeply, focusing, or relaxing. OM Yoga Center founder Cyndi Lee calls it a "calm abiding" that comes from the noble serenity of a "Buddha Mind."[12] Of course one need not be a Buddhist to practice meditation and enjoy its many benefits. The idea is that anyone can learn to train the mind to deal more successfully with the vicissitudes of life, from daily stress to the anxiety of a Broadway audition or a Carnegie Hall debut. Lee espouses the meditative practice *Shamatha* as a means of accessing a Buddha Mind instead of the mind of a panicked antelope running for its life while being chased by a ferocious lion.

*Shamatha practice is a technique for staying centered within our evolving world. It's not about creating an unmoving blissful state, but about having the courage to experience all the states of mind that arise and pass, just like weather…When we can begin to stop wishing things were different and learn to ride movement, we will shift toward a state of balance, of unconditional contentment.*[13]

Shamatha involves being in the moment, living and doing your best performance at that moment. Often singers are instead focused on what just went wrong onstage while they are still onstage performing. Instead of staying in the moment and committed to the performance still taking place, they become distracted by the recent past, berating themselves for any memory slips, musical errors, or perceived imperfections in their sound. Or they may agonize about potential pitfalls that they may encounter, for instance worrying about high notes that might falter, which often causes them to falter. The typical physical and psychological manifestations of stage fright rob the singer of confidence and thus hinder his/her ability to realize and display his/her true talent and potential. In this sense, singers are akin to athletes who need a positive mental outlook so their body can perform positively. The inner monologue of Paul Bettany in the film *Wimbledon* ("Don't choke! Please don't choke!") sheds light on the athlete's struggle with negative thinking and fear of failure. It is reminiscent of Carolyn Leigh's lyrics from the Broadway musical *Peter Pan*, in which Peter coaches Michael Darling on flying by advising, "Lovelier thoughts, Michael." It's simple sports psychology, but somehow it's never quite that simple.

## BACKSTAGE YOGA

When directing an opera, I lead my cast through a pre-show yoga warm-up, emphasizing rib-opening poses like Gate and Triangle as well as asanas to energize the body (Warrior Two), focus the mind (Tree), and calm performance anxiety (Lotus). For myself, I do Ujjayi breathing backstage to slow and control my breath when nerves start my heart racing. Mantra meditation between sets during a recital helps me stay centered on the text I need to remember and brings calm and confidence to my psyche which I can take onstage with me.

In the insightful book *Power Performance for Singers*, voice teacher Shirlee Emmons teamed with sports psychologist Alma Thomas to investigate what empowers singers to perform at their best. In their estimation, a peak performance is facilitated by the presence of the following elements: no feelings of fear, an ability to regulate anxiety and arousal, maintenance of positive thoughts and imagery, high confidence, an ability to remain focused and concentrated, determination to succeed, thinking that is committed and disciplined, and control over the performance.[14]

Of course there is no perfect performance, and no one ever has complete control onstage. There are too many variables in live performance for it ever to be "perfect," but the magic and risk of performing live are (or should be) a thrill for performers and audience alike. With proper preparation, rehearsal, and technique, singers should be able to perform with consistency and creativity as long as they can come to grips with managing performance anxiety. Meditation endows the singer with a mode of setting up and sustaining the emotional and physical balance necessary so that performing is a pleasurable and positive event that enlightens artistry instead of obscuring it.

Optimism, positivism and Pollyanna have long been a part of the American mindset. From Little Orphan Annie comics during the Depression (we'll avoid discussion of the obvious, overly familiar and redundant *Annie* song) to Norman Vincent Peale's 1957 book *The Power of Positive Thinking*, we have been told that sanguine confidence leads to success à la *The Little Engine That Could*: "I know I can! I know I can!" In more recent times, the eloquent and incredibly prolific Deepak Chopra has written multiple books on empowering the mind, body, and spirit. With his combined knowledge of and interest in both medicine and meditation, Chopra brought accessibility and legitimacy to the power of (and need for) meditation in contemporary Western life. Motivational speakers and authors such as Wayne Dyer (*Being in Balance* and *Change Your Thoughts, Change Your Life: Living the Wisdom of the Tao*) have taken the concept even more into the mainstream. We are not talking about transcendental meditation (TM), the search for nirvana, Samadhi or a state of divine bliss. We don't want to transcend the body, because as singers it is our unique, essential, and sole instrument. And we don't want to transcend the mind entirely, because we need to remember the words we are supposed to sing. Instead we are trying to transcend topophobia (the fancy word for stage fright), seeking a way to realize a performance that is "in the zone" as opposed to in the midst of the racing heartbeat, clammy hands, and cotton mouth of stage fright.

# COUNTRY DUO SUGARLAND AND "SHOW-GA"

Singer **Jennifer Nettles** and background vocalist/guitarist **Kristian Bush** talked with CMT about the benefits yoga brings to their singing and performing.

**Bush**: I have always heard that über-successful people who write books about how to become über-successful all have one thing in common: they all meditate every day. I consider yoga my meditation.

**Nettles**: The actual purpose of yoga is to prepare the body and mind for meditation. I love the feeling of space and calm that comes after a practice. The distractions of the day have been left behind when you step on the mat so that when you step off, you are more fully yourself. It is a beautiful feeling. The most relaxed you could ever feel. The idea that life and work has a flow and we would all benefit from not pushing too

hard within that flow is so helpful. The conscious awareness of your body and emotional state is helpful, too, in learning when to pause or take a moment for yourself before moving forward with a show.

**Bush**: We are always experimenting with our show. I think we were just having fun naturally playing off each other on stage one day and did backbends facing each other. It really became "show-ga" as soon as Jennifer made up a name for it.

**Nettles**: Show-ga is actually moments where we incorporate some yoga elements into our physical show. You could see backbends or triangle pose. You never know.

*"The last three days of shooting I was in the Lotus position. And the Lotus position took me fourteen months to get. I did an hour and a half a day of yoga to be able to get there."*

—*Hugh Jackman*
*(Tony Award-winner for the musical "The Boy from Oz") did yoga in the film "The Fountain" (2006)*

# Dharana: Focus

Singing involves a high level of physical and mental coordination. You don't want to sing with unnecessary tension but at the same time you should not be relaxed or lax onstage. Instead, you should be alert and attentive without being anxious or angst-ridden.

The supreme goal should be, in a word, **focus**. Singers work hard to learn to focus their voices, to create a clear, focused sound with balanced resonance. But often they are not taught to focus their minds as well in order to find clarity of thinking and emotional balance. The initial step of deep meditation, Dharana, is about focusing the mind and maintaining or holding concentration (ekagrata). There are so many distractions that prevent our minds from staying focused even when we are singing in front of audience. The frantic pace of modern life plus the proliferation of multi-tasking and Attention Deficit Disorder (ADD) contribute to the diffusion of mental focus. Add the doubts and fears brought on by nervous apprehension and the brain begins to write its own cadenza of *agitato*, staccato thoughts. As Iyengar observes, "the mind is an instrument, the product of thoughts which are difficult to restrain for they are subtle and fickle."[15] To rewrite the famous Verdi aria from *Rigoletto*, it's not "La donna" but "La mente" or the mind which "è mobile."

In order to contend with the seemingly moveable and unsettled state of the mind, you must become mindful, and not critical of the body. You should cultivate awareness and alertness centered on a single mental focal point. Banish unnecessary thoughts. Meditation is and should be a highly personal act. Only you can know what will work for you. Dhyana or meditation is usually done in Bound Angle, Lotus, or Corpse pose, but you can do it standing backstage or sitting in your dressing room chair. Close your eyes, perhaps dim the lights, and begin to focus inward. As you try to focus your mind, focus on your breath by taking long, slow inhalations. Use the Kala pranayama technique to lengthen and equalize the breath cycle. Breath control plays an integral role in calming the mind and body during meditation. The Kundalini school avers, "the effect of rhythmic breathing in inducing changes in brainwave pattern is well known. If you slow the breath to eight breaths per minute you move into a meditative state; slow the rhythm to six breaths and the pituitary gland is stimulated."[16] By stimulating the pituitary gland, this meditation supposedly unblocks the so-called third eye, bringing focus, clarity, and inner vision. Eight breaths a minute may seem daunting at first, but don't panic. If you inhale for 4 counts and exhale for 4 counts, then that is roughly eight breaths a minute. A rate of six breaths per minute is about 5 counts of inhalation and 5 counts of exhalation. Just as you wouldn't expect to traverse long Straussian or Wagnerian phrases overnight, you shouldn't expect to control your breath rate overnight. Practice and be patient with yourself, just as you should with your singing.

# Mantras

Mantras are a common means of focusing the mind during meditation. Mantra [mantra] means "mind deliverance," thus a mantra is an instrument of thought that helps to deliver or liberate the mind. More simply, a mantra is a self-affirming word or phrase that is meant to be repeated (either audibly or internally) in order to bring self-assurance. In even simpler terms, it's a personal pep talk. Cathy in Jason Robert Brown's *The Last Five Years* appears to be somewhat well-versed in mantras, using them to quell her fears during her audition in "Climbing Uphill." Despite the quality of her mantras ("I am a good person, I am an attractive person, I am a talented person: grant me grace"), unfortunately she does not focus single-mindedly and thus is unable to dispel her doubt ("I suck").

Mantra yoga, known in Sanskrit as Japa yoga (meaning to utter in a low voice) can utilize an audible repetition, as will be explored in Chapter 5 on Chanting, or an unspoken repetition within the mind. For our purposes, pick a mental mantra, a silent self-heartening slogan that you will repeat internally. A number of song titles provide inspiration and ideas for mantras, such as Finch's "I Believe in You" from *How to Succeed in Business Without Really Trying*, Jekyll and Hyde's "This is the Moment," and Gloria Gaynor's disco classic "I Will Survive." Rosina's aria "Una voce poco fa" from *The Barber of Seville* is replete with confidence boosting repetitions of "vincerò" (I will win!), as is the climatic ending of Calaf's aria "Nessun dorma" from *Turandot*. Also chock full of positive pronouncements are the lyrics of Helen Reddy's familiar feminist anthem: "I am strong, I am invincible, I am Woman." Other inspiring mantras include "I Can Go the Distance" of Disney's *Hercules*, and the moving protest song and civil rights anthem "We Shall Overcome." But my favorite mantra-like lyric has to be Maria von Trapp's in *The Sound of Music*: "I have confidence in me."

While a mantra is highly personal, choose it carefully. If you wish, God may be part of your mantra or it may be spiritual in a less specific way, for there can certainly be a prayer-like aspect to a mantra. Make sure it is assertive and substantially affirming. For instance, Sally Bowles in *Cabaret* sets herself up for failure with the low expectations of "Maybe This Time." Instead, follow *Funny Girl* Fanny Brice's mantra as a model: "I'm the Greatest Star!" You can change your mantra daily or weekly as befits your current mental outlook, but there is an advantage to the familiarity of a consistently used mantra, just as there is comfort and assurance in a habitual vocal warm-up or pre-performance routine. The mental echo of the mantra in your mind can block out a negative inner monologue and has a calming and hypnotic effect on the body. The length of your mantra is also up to you, but it should not last longer than a comfortable exhalation and should not get too complicated. Remember the power and focus of simplicity.

Here are some mantras that have been helpful to me and my students. These are not necessarily suggestions (although feel free to use them since there is no copyright on silent mantras!) but they may also be used as a springboard for finding your own preferred and personalized mantras.

## SOME SECULAR MANTRAS

*I will sing at my best. I am in control. I can do this.*
*I am at peace. My spirit will soar.*

*I center myself in stillness and trust. My talent will shine.*
*I will make my dreams come true.*

## SOME MORE SPIRITUAL MANTRAS

*I am blessed by the love of God. God is with me.*
*I greet this day with confidence and faith.*

*I know the abundant love of God fills my life with good.*
*The Holy Spirit sings in me.*

In her book *Creative Visualization*, Shakti Gawain provides some valuable guidelines for mantras or affirmations. She stresses the importance of phrasing affirmations "in the present tense, not in the future."[17] Theoretically this helps to actualize the thoughts instead of thinking of them merely as potential energy. But do what works for you. Sometimes I find great strength and comfort in affirming thoughts of the future. Of her principles regarding affirmations, the following seem of particular relevance:

• Always phrase affirmations in the most positive way you can. Affirm what you do want, not what you don't.

• In general, the shorter and simpler your affirmation, the more effective it is.

• Try as much as possible to create a feeling of belief; experience that your affirmations can be true.[18]

However you choose to construct or phrase your mantras, use the power of mantra in your meditation by finding comfort in the ritual and repetition and in the power of positive thinking.

*17, 18* From *Creative Visualization*. Copyright © 2002 by Shakti Gawain. Reprinted with permission of New World Library, Novato, CA. www.newworldlibrary.com

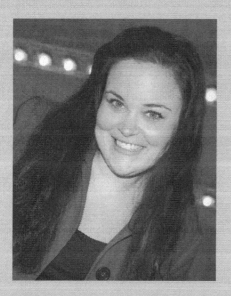

I believe yoga and meditation are essential to singing and performing. I have made great vocal strides simply from singing a song entirely in Downward Dog. Weird? Yes. Extremely helpful? Absolutely! I have found incorporating yoga into my singing practice allows me to take my mind off of the "technique" and puts the tension somewhere other than my throat, making me sing with greater ease. Suddenly belting high Es and Fs is a piece of cake.

The mental aspect of yoga is possibly my favorite. I have terrible stage fright, but after doing a few yoga poses and deep breaths and incorporating positive thinking into my warm-ups, those nerves are not nearly as intense. This is extremely helpful during auditions! Basically, yoga has changed my life.

*–Jessica Miesel,*
*BFA in Musical Theatre,*
*former featured singer with*
*Texas Legacies*

# Mudras

Mantras may be used as the primary component in your meditation or you may use them in combination with mudras. Meaning "seal" in Sanskrit, a mudra [mu'dra] is a symbolic hand gesture that can be used to direct and deepen meditation. Although you can do many mudras while standing or lying down, they are most often done in a seated position. As you sit in Easy pose or Lotus, adopt one of the following hand positions, choosing the mudra which seems most in line with your mantra and mindset. You can hold the mudra anywhere from 3 minutes to a half hour, whatever time you need to feel its influence. Remarkably, the hand movements and postures impact other parts of the body. These effects are enumerated by Swiss yogi Gertrud Hirschi:

*There is a direct relationship between the hands and the neck since the nerve paths run through the vertebral foramina in the arms, hands, and fingers. The flexibility of the hands always effects [sic] the flexibility of the neck, therefore hand exercises relieve tensions in the neck. Moreover, spreading the ten fingers creates a reflex that causes the thoracic (chest) vertebrae to spread out. This increases the tidal volume of the lungs. The hands and/ or fingers also have an additional direct relationship to the heart and lungs...[A] crooked hand position also impedes inhalation. The result is that the optimum amount of air is not drawn into the lungs.[19]*

The importance of optimal lung capacity and an unimpeded inhalation needs little explanation. Obviously singers can only benefit from a free and flexible neck, since rigidity in the neck will cause tension in the ever-important larynx. You need not subscribe to acupressure, reflexology, or palmistry to profit from employing mudras in your meditation. So realize the power of mudras to seal, settle, and strengthen your meditation.

## NAMASTE OR PRAYER MUDRA [namas'de]

This hand position should already be familiar from the prayer twist asanas. Center your practice in this mudra because it provides a good starting and ending point for your meditation.

- Hold each hand with the fingers together.
- Place the palms together as if in prayer.
- Maintaining the prayer position, bring your hands closer to the body to rest gently on the chest.

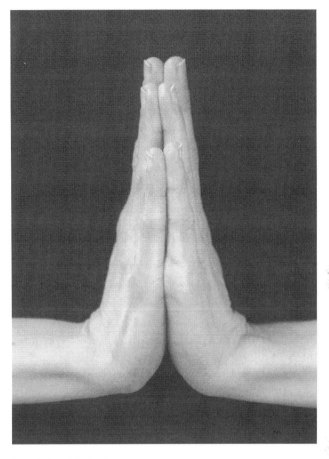

"En prière" –Gabriel Fauré

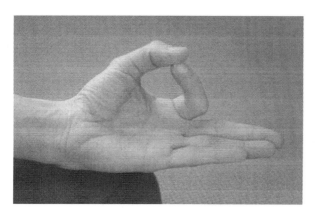

"I Concentrate on You." –Cole Porter

## JNANA MUDRA ['djana]

Probably the best-known meditative gesture, this mudra sharpens memory and concentration, which makes it a great pre-performance mudra for those worried about forgetting song texts or vocal entrances.

- Sit in Lotus.
- With each hand, bend the index finger and bring it to the middle of the top phalange of your thumb (the fleshy tip).
- Extend the other fingers and gently rest the back of the the wrists on the knees.

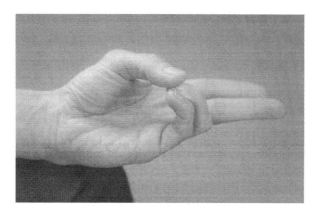

"The House of Life." –Ralph Vaughan Williams

## PRANA MUDRA ['prana]

Remember prana is energy or life, so this mudra increases energy, vitality, and confidence if you are feeling un-energized and/or unsure before an audition.

- With each hand resting palms upward on your knees, touch your thumb to the tips of your ring and pinkie fingers.
- Keep the other fingers (middle and index) extended and facing upwards (like the peace sign, but with the middle and index fingers touching instead of spread into a V).
- Hold as you rest the backs of the wrists on the knees.

# APANA MUDRA [a'pana]

Ground yourself with this balancing mudra if performance anxiety has you feeling out of control.

• With each hand, bring your thumb together with the tips of your middle and ring fingers.
• Keep the other fingers (pinkie and index) extended upwards (like "I love you" in sign language).
• Hold as you rest the backs of the wrists on the knees.

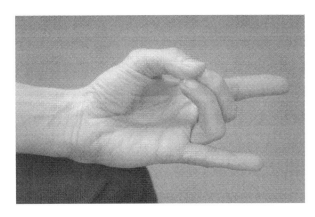

"Solid Ground." –Coldplay

# MATANGI MUDRA [ma'taŋgi]

This mudra is inspired by Matangi, the god of inner harmony. This multipurpose posture brings a sense of calm, strengthens expansion at the solar plexus, and helps relieve jaw tension via a reflexology/pressure point (a particularly wonderful benefit for many singers with jaw issues).

• Interlace your fingers as you hold your hands in front of the solar plexus.
• Unite and extend the middle fingers outwards as your press them together isometrically.

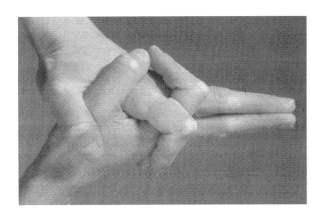

"The Praise of Harmony." –Handel's *Alexander's Feast*

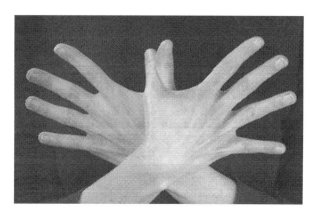

Mendelssohn's "Auf Flügeln des Gesanges" (On the Wings of Song)

# GARUDA MUDRA ['garuda]

Associated with respiration, this "mystical bird" or eagle mudra soothes mood fluctuations and stimulates circulation so your spirit can take flight in song.

• With your palms in front of you facing the body, cross the hands and interlace the thumbs as you spread the fingers like the wings of a bird.
• Begin with your hands in front of your lower abdomen.
• In cycles of ten breaths, repeat with the hands at the navel, then at the solar plexus, and finally at the sternum.

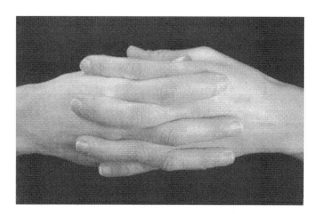

"He's got the whole world in his hands." –Traditional spiritual

# USHAS MUDRA ['uʃas]

Known as the origin of all good things, this "break of day" or sunrise mudra is particularly good for morning meditation. It also relates to creativity and new beginnings, so it can bring energy to rehearsing a new song or aria.

• With your palms facing you, clasp and interlace the fingers with the thumbs pressing together. (Supposedly men should have the right thumb on top while women should have the left on top.)

# GANESHA MUDRA
# [gaˈneʃa]

Named after the elephant deity Ganesh, this mudra is about overcoming obstacles. Try this mudra to help combat vocal or musical challenges.

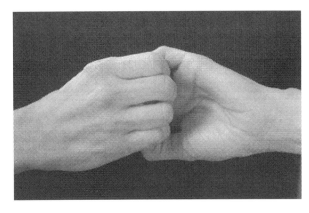

"Let those eyes sparkle and shine." –*Dumbo*'s mother

- With your left hand in front of the chest and the left palm facing away from the body, bend the fingers and grasp the right hand with the right palm facing the body.
- Bring the hands in front of the chest.
- As you exhale, grip and pull the hands apart without releasing the fingers.
- Then inhale and release the tension without releasing the hands.
- Repeat with the right palm facing outward and the left palm facing inward.
- This mudra may be done with the arm horizontal or diagonal as desired.

In promotional pictures for her album *Bionic* (2010), pop diva Christina Aguilera posed doing the mind-centering Chi mudra (like Jnana mudra except the thumb and index finger round without actually touching).

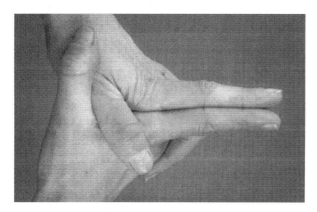

"Enlighten me." –Echo and the Bunnymen

## UTTARABODHI MUDRA [uʻtarabodi]

Considered the mudra of highest enlightenment, this hand position strengthens inhalation and provides energy and inspiration. Therefore it is ideal before a big singing debut performance.

• Fold both hands in front of the solar plexus.
• Join and extend the index fingers against each other and the thumbs against each other.

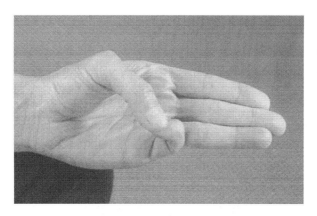

"Let it Flow." –Toni Braxton

## BHUDI MUDRA [ʻbudi]

This mudra helps to maintain the body's fluid balance and to ameliorate dry mouth, which oftens plagues nervous singers.

• With each hand, join the tip of the thumb and pinkie finger.
• Extend the three middle fingers and gently rest the wrists on the knees.

Explore mudras and/or mantras as meditative tools. Use meditation to focus your mind, to reduce stress, to awaken creativity, or to bring a sense of peace to your life and to your singing. In *The Inner Game of Music*, symphonic musician Barry Green draws some interesting parallels between musical dissonance and the mental discord of life:

> *Most Western music is based on a harmonic system of creating and resolving dissonance. Effectively, this means that the music gains its power from setting up musical tensions and stresses, and then resolving them...in serene and harmonious endings...When we realize that what at first looks like a stressful or negative experience can be understood as a "dissonance" that can lead to resolution, we can begin to accept the stressful moments and flow with them instead of resisting them.*[20]

Green's outlook echoes Cyndi Lee's and brings us back to the practice of Shamatha.

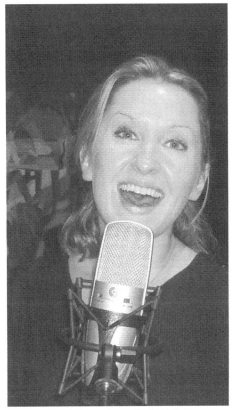

The bhudi mudra helps my dry mouth after all that "Black Coffee." —Emily Gail, jazz vocalist

We cannot necessarily avoid the ups and downs of life, the unpredictability of live performance or the trepidation of imperfection, bad reviews, or perceived failure. But meditation can bestow the concentration and confidence we need as singers to quiet the inner demons of doubt, to maximize our ability to sing with focus and freedom, and to reduce the pressure while you rediscover and reclaim the pleasure of performing.

# 5

# Sound Yoga: Chanting and Musical Meditation

*"Chant and be happy."*

— George Harrison

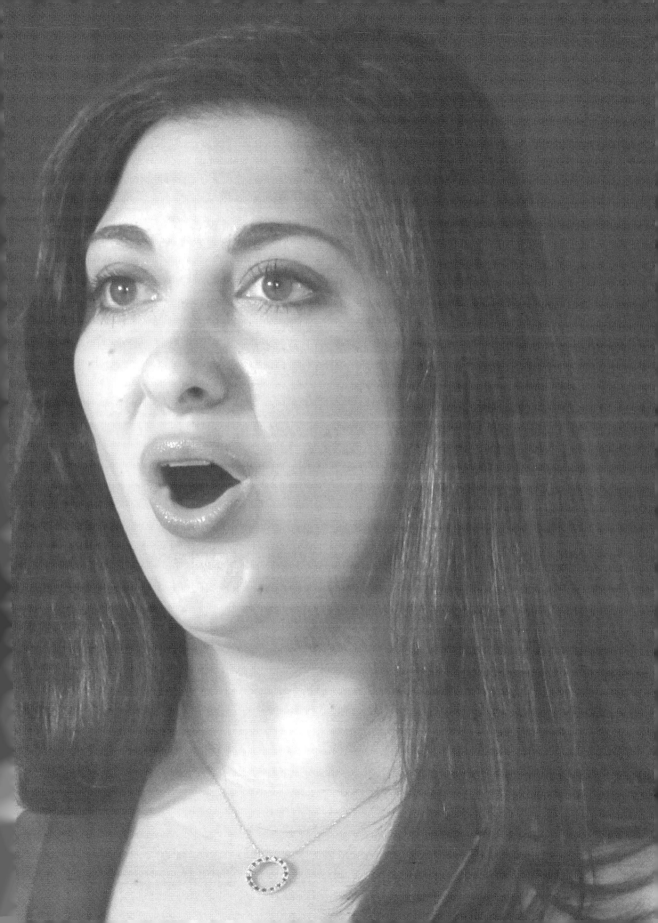

*"As I watch Alanis perform, it strikes me, this is ritual, she is dervish-whirling; she is chanting, lyrical chants about the emotional world and daily life experience.*
*This whole thing is ritual for her, she's practicing her yoga by performing."*

— **Wade Imre Morissette**,
*yoga teacher and Alanis Morissette's twin brother, LA Yoga magazine, December 2008/January 2009*

Since chanting involves the voice, it is an obvious means of attracting singers to exploring and excelling at meditation. The purpose of examining chant is not for stylistic reasons or for discovering new repertoire. There are Vedic chant-like passages in Phillip Glass's minimalist Sanskrit opera *Satyagraha*, and raga-grounded melodies may be found throughout India's Bollywood movie musicals, the West End/Broadway musical *Bombay Dreams*, or the Academy Award-winning film *Slumdog Millionaire*. But chanting is a means to an end, a method to heighten meditation by amplifying focus via vocal vibration. In silent meditation, your mantra still resonates in your mind and thus emanates throughout the body. But verbalizing or voicing the mantra aloud adds tangible, visceral resonance which can magnify meditation's calming and centering properties.

*Contemporary medical research has shown that chanting and other forms of vocalization actually oxygenate the cells, lower blood pressure and heart rate, increase lymphatic circulation increase levels of melatonin, reduce stress-related hormones, release endorphins (the body's natural painkillers)...Vocal sound is proving itself to be a vibrant healing energy.*[21]

No wonder we singers love to sing! The vibration of your own voice can have a massage-like effect on the body, perhaps reminding us of the vibratory sensations of our mother's voice when we were in womb.

# Shabda Yoga: Say OM

Shabda or word yoga literally gives a voice to the union of mind and body. Mantras are verbalized or vocalized, spoken or sung in a repetitive concentration technique which calms and focuses a restless mind through chant's rhythmic, mesmerizing capabilities. The mantra reverberates through the body, a process enhanced by chanting in a group setting or chanting back to back with a partner. The most commonly chanted mantra is Om [aum]. This Sanskrit word shares a linguistic root meaning with the Latin word Omne, which means all. Om embodies the sound of all sounds, the sound of the universe. Although it is a single syllable, Om is comprised of three separate sounds. Each should be intoned in an elongated manner on a single, extended exhalation. These three sounds possess multiple symbolic meanings singly and as a unit:

| IPA symbol | Time Symbol | Yoga Symbol | Symbol of Consciousness | Mantra Symbol |
|---|---|---|---|---|
| [a] | past | asana | conscious/ waking state | That |
| [u] | present | pranayama | dream state | Thou |
| [m] | future | pratyahara | dreamless sleep state | Art |
| [aum] | universe | samadhi | transcendent state | One |

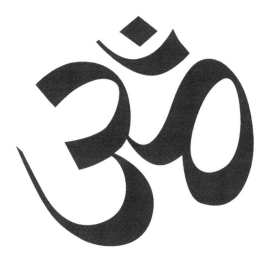

# OM and More

The most universally known mantra is Om, which happens to symbol-ize the universe. Om is a sacred sound or syllable for Hinduism, Bud-dhism and Jainism. The Sanskrit symbol for Om has begun to enter the symbology of Western culture, in part due to its relevance to yoga and meditation. It is interesting to note the similarity of Om to holy words or prayerful expressions from other languages and religions: Amen or אָמֵן in Hebrew (Judaism and Christianity), Amin آمين, (Ara-bic), Omne (Latin), Omnipotent (English), and Omega Ω (Greek).

With its three sounds, OM or AUM evokes other tripartite religious ritual and symbolism. According to the Talmud, a status of perma-nence is established when an event repeats itself three times. There are three iterations of Sanctus (Holy) within the Ordinary of the Mass. In the Eastern Orthodox liturgy, a three-part responsorial Alleluia is sung. And OM is often chanted three times at the beginning and the end of a yoga class to bring balance, focus, and strength to the practice.

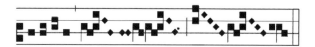

Alleluia

The Om symbol in Tamil makes me think of the elephant Ganesh.

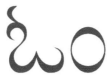

The swan-like Om symbol in Kannada, Telugu, and Tulu.

The symbol for Omkar in Bengali seems to evoke Lotus position.

The curving arcs of Om in Balinese remind me of Reverse Warrior pose.

The Tibetan Om is a complex symbol with images of ascension.

Om in Jain script almost suggests Locust pose.

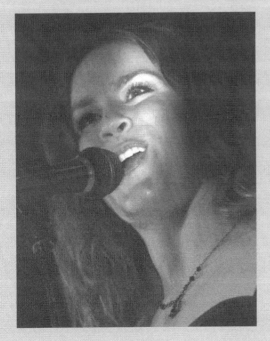

When practiced with awareness, yoga can bring one more into vibrational alignment. It allows a person to vibrate higher, which in turn allows dreams and desires to come to fruition. Source energy can be expressed more freely without the barriers we put up, and yoga is about unbinding and dissolving barriers (spiritual and physical) that we have built through accumulated negative emotion in our lives. To be un-bound, to be free...what could be more helpful in allowing our dreams to come true? What could be more helpful in preparing for a performance? In embodying a character? In allowing deep, full breath? In enabling unencumbered movement and posture? Yoga is a powerful way for any performer to tap into the tremendous potential that lies beneath the surface levels!

*–Sarah Strable, lead singer of Black and Blue*

From a purely vocal viewpoint, Om can be a useful exercise since it combines the central lingual or tongue vowel [a] with the back labial or lip vowel [u] and the bi-labial nasal hum [m]. Thus even without any symbolic or spiritual implications, Om can be helpful in creating awareness of vowel formation and vocal production as well as resonance alignment or keeping the placement of your voice consistent.

Chant is usually performed on a series of one, two or three repeated pitches known as reciting tones. Nada or sound yoga specialist Russill Paul provides helpful guidelines on selecting pitches for ideal resonance in your chanting.

*The base tone is the default pitch. It should be centered in the heart... [and] resonates in the mid-chest. A high tone is to be used above the base tone, and a low tone below it; this causes the energy of the mantra to move up into the head and belly, alternating between these three centers...The power of moving among three tones sustains the wavelength of sound frequencies generated by our brain, streamlining our mental processes toward the intention of the mantra.*[22]

*"I prepare mentally by listening to my mantra chant 'om namah shivaya' as a devotion of Siddha yoga. Performing is very spiritual for me. I do meditation--I try to eat light and well, get enough sleep, come from a place of gratitude, warm up very lightly and commit to giving my all every show I do."*

—**Ann Hampton Callaway**, *cabaret singer sharing her pre-show ritual on broadway.com*

22 From *The Yoga of Sound*. Copyright © 2004 by Russill Paul. Reprinted with permission of New World Library, Novato, CA. www.newworldlibrary.com

With chant novices, I will often play music dominated by a drone or repeated, prolonged pitch. Singers will easily match the base tone, better known to them as the tonic or "do." Playing a drone that is an open fifth (the tonic and fifth, or do and sol) can create the centering effect thanks to the symmetry and purity of this perfect interval. The goal is not to sing both pitches at once like the throat singers of Tuva. That would be diplophonia, which is considered a vocal fault in Western music. The purpose of having the group sing in unison, octaves or fifths is not about creating a choral blend but to encourage tuning of minds and spirits to bring a sense of community harmony. This exercise can be particularly helpful for creating a feeling of ensemble within a cast near the beginning of the rehearsal period or during warm-ups before a performance.

While Om is universally used and recognized, there are certainly many other possible mantras for chanting. Instead of chanting in Sanskrit, you could choose an English mantra. Avoid words that end in a plosive consonant such as [ b ], [ p ], [ k ], [ g ], [ d ], or [ t ]. It is beneficial to have a continuant consonant if there is a final consonant to the word because this encourages continuing vibrations conducive to chant. You may wish to chant an English word which holds more personal or emotional significance. Here are some monosyllabic English words which might be good mantras, obviously because of their meaning but also because of their phonetic components.

## PEACE [pis]

The [i] vowel is a good focal point and the sibilant [s] encourages long, steady exhalation.

## JOY [dʒoi]

The opening voiced affricate is vitalizing and the diphthong of [oi] nurtures balance between back and frontal vowels.

## CALM [kam]

The combination of the central [a] vowel and the bi-labial hum can recreate the calm of the original Om.

## LOVE [lʌv]

The liquid [l] leads into a neutral central vowel and finishes with the wonderful vibratory sensation of the fricative [v].

## BE [bi]

After the energizing initial [b], this mantra is all about sustaining the highly focused [i] vowel.

Multi-syllabic mantras are not common but they can still work. An obvious choice for an English mantra in this vein would be Amen. In addition to its familiar religious overtones, Amen provides two nasal continuants for easy, resonant humming. For a more complex Sanskrit mantra, you could try Om shanti. Shanti [ʃanti] means peace, so this mantra personifies universal peace, a wonderful and unifying concept on which to chant and meditate.

# Toning:
# Vowels and Humming

Chant need not, however, employ actual words. Vocalizing on a single extended vowel sound, called toning, allows you to focus very single-mindedly
on one sound. Thus it can certainly help bring the mind to a single focus. In
addition to bolstering concentration, toning spotlights a single vowel sound,
thereby compelling the singer to concentrate on the quality or timbre and
resonance of the vowel. It is similar to the long tones often employed by wind
players at the beginning of their practice. Toning heightens awareness of the
rate of air flow and vibrato, helping to steady and equalize both. Furthermore, toning affords the opportunity to work on dynamic control. Akin to the
technique of *messa di voce* espoused by vocal pedagogue Manuel Garcia II
(1805-1906), toning can include the steady crescendo and decrescendo on a
single pitch which defines this expressive musical device. Thus it appears that
toning can have positive effects on both technique and musicality, enhancing
the quality of the singer's sound and expression.

## CELEBRITY YOGIS:

Singer/actress **Shirley MacLaine** is a long-time yoga devotee. Her
video *Inner Workout: A Program for Relaxation and Stress Reduction
through Meditation* (1989) includes guided chakra meditation through
color imagery to help you find "that wonderful feeling of knowing your
own power."

**Barbra Streisand** reportedly used chanting and meditation to help
overcome the performance anxiety which kept her off the concert
stage for 27 years.

*"The most interesting aspect about the calm center of a singer is that it is a volcano. It is a burning, engaged core, which ignites when you want it to ignite for the purpose you choose. Some yoga teachers actually refer to stillness as not being still."*

— **Thomas Hampton**, *baritone,*
*Classical Singer magazine,*
*October 2003*

In order to maintain balance, it is advisable to tone on all of the vowels. However, most singers have a predilection for certain vowel sounds and aversions to others. No doubt these preferences will impact your choice of vowels when chanting, but explore the varying properties and effects of the vowels. With their highly focused and frontal resonance, the front vowels [i] and [e] are clarifying and vitalizing. They create a strong vibratory sensation on the hard palate/roof of the mouth due to the high, arched position of the front part of the body of the tongue. The central vowel [a] can be a centering point, thanks to its flat tongue and open mouth position. Although it is the most common vowel for vocalises, cadenzas and coloratura, the proper position for [a] can be difficult for some singers to find. So that [a] does not feel like no man's land, it can be advantageous to begin toning from [i] to [a] and back to [i] to create kinesthetic awareness of the tongue position needed for accurate vowel formation. Due to their lip-rounding and thus lengthening of the vocal tract, the labial vowels [o] and [u] can have a highly soothing effect. These back vowels create a sense of space in the back of the mouth and encourage one to turn inward for the introspection of meditation. Finally, humming is a good way to ease the uncertain initiates into chanting. The bi-labial [m] fosters muscle memory of frontal vocal placement since the focal point of the sound is the closed lips. Similarly, the velar hum [ŋ] helps promote head voice resonance in the masque and promotes perception of the position of the elusive soft palate. Tone on these vowels and/ or hum on the nasal continuants either alone or in combinations that make sense to you and your vocal and meditative issues.

If you wish to delve into kundalini concepts in greater detail, you can explore the relation of certain vowels to the seven chakras or wheels of energy. Energy is thought to emanate and vibrate through these seven meridians in the body as defined by the chakras. The fifth through seventh chakras are of most relevance to singers. The throat chakra is important to singers for obvious reasons since it involves sound, self-expression, and the voice itself. But also of interest are the sixth chakra, the so-called third eye or brow chakra which is particularly associated with chanting Om, and the seventh or the crown chakra, as it relates to meditation.

# MUSIC FOR YOGA

Singers are musicians of course, so music is usually an integral and inspiring part of their yoga practice. Music can help set a serene mood, focus the mind, and even calm the body and spirit with trance-like, repetitive music. Think of World Music (particularly Indian or African), new age music (Enya, Kitaro, George Winston) or of classical composers exploring minimalism such as Phillip Glass, Steve Reich, or John Tavener. Some of my favorites include Henryk Mikołaj Górecki's *Symphony of Sorrowful Songs* or *The Prayer Cycle* by Jonathan Elias (featuring singers such as James Taylor and Alanis Morissette). I also enjoy practicing yoga to the music of Lilith Fair founder Sarah McLachlan, herself a yogi. Others may prefer to practice in silence, or to the music of nature. Few things are more amazing than doing Sun Salutations at sunrise on the beach, to the soothing sound of waves lapping on the sand.

Here are some of the associations between the chakras, vocal sounds, notes of the musical scale, and even colors and states of mind.

| Chakra number | Chakra center | Sound (in IPA) | Pitch/Solfege Symbol | Keyword | Color |
|---|---|---|---|---|---|
| 1st | Root | [o] | Do | Grounding | Red |
| 2nd | Sacral | [u] | Re | Creativity | Orange |
| 3rd | Navel | [a] | Mi | Power | Yellow |
| 4th | Heart | [e] | Fa | Compassion | Green |
| 5th | Throat | [i] | Sol | Communication | Blue |
| 6th | Third Eye | [m] | La | Intuition | Indigo |
| 7th | Crown | [ŋ] | Ti | Acceptance | Violet |

For advanced kundalini chanting with chakra work, you could coordinate your toning on these specific sounds and pitches to nurture balance and alignment of energy through the meridians of the body. For instance, to foster creativity, intone the [u] vowel on Re (D in C major) while picturing an orange wheel of energy emanating from and encircling the lower back. For some, these techniques may become too intricate or seem too convoluted. But you can experiment to see what works for you as you explore how toning can aid in aligning and harmonizing the voice, body, mind, and spirit.

Entailing a number of methods which relate musical pitch to pranayama, sound yoga brings a practical and tangible application of yoga to singing. Chanting on mantras and toning vowels reveal numerous benefits, from the soothing effects of sound therapy or music therapy to increased awareness of acoustic phonetics and vocal harmonics. Not only does chanting integrate yoga practices directly to your singing by giving a vocal and musical element to meditation, it presents some ways to improve vowel production and resonance and thereby strengthen your vocal technique. So, as Beatle George Harrison advised in his album title, "Chant and be happy" because of the manifold benefits of uniting voice, breath, and body in sonic meditation.

*"I think only about going onstage and singing well. It is very difficult for the nerves. I have to control it, like yoga, to have the concentration to be very relaxed."*

—**Roberto Alagna**, *tenor, Opera News, October 2001*

# Conclusion: Bringing Yoga to Life in Your Life

*"Yoga is 99% practice."*

Sri Krishna Pattabhi Jois

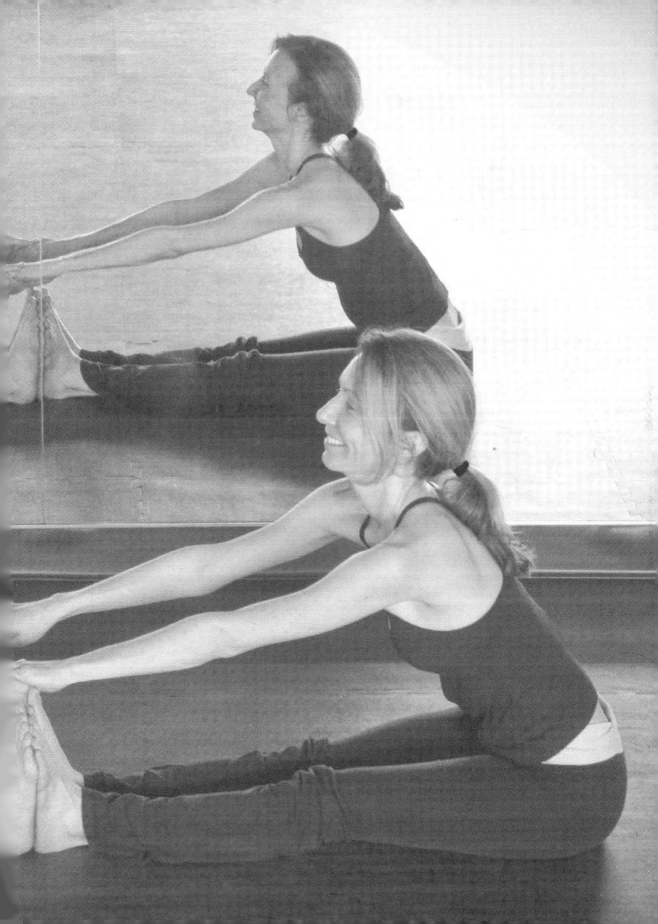

In music, they say practice makes perfect. In truth, and in real life, perfection does not exist. But practice does make better and as with singing, practicing yoga is the path to improvement, enjoyment, and development of your skills. Of course you should check with your doctor before beginning any new exercise program, and certain health issues (such as knee or back problems, high blood pressure, and pregnancy) need to be taken into consideration. But find the way that yoga can be part of your life. Regardless of your health, size, weight, experience level or comfort level, yoga can help you with the physical and emotional challenges of your life on and off the stage. Finding a yoga class is not difficult anymore. There is a proliferation of yoga classes available now, at gyms, colleges, yoga centers and dance studios. Ideally you would begin your yoga work with a teacher to guide you in person. But if that is not an option, then a number of fine yoga DVDs are available that can get you started and still provide a model for form and reinforcement of important concepts. The series by Yoga Journal is particularly good, featuring great yoga teachers such as Patricia Walden and Rodney Yee. There are also a number of free yoga podcasts.

Perhaps a few asanas can be part of your morning routine, or the breathing techniques of pranayama could precede and lead into your vocal warm-up. Vinyasas and/or toning could be incorporated into a group warm-up before a show or concert to unify a cast of diverse performers, energies, and egos. Moreover, yoga provides a powerful method in coping with performance anxiety. Some musicians have turned to beta blockers or Xanax to deal with the stress of stage fright, but yoga proves there is a medication-free, self-nurturing method of combating the pressure of performing. Explore the different schools and styles of yoga to see which fits you best. Whether it is in the empowering flow of a Warrior series vinyasa, the serene strength of sustaining a single asana, the quiet calm of silent solo meditation or the spiritual group setting of chanting mantras, yoga grants concrete ways to focus the mind, calm the nerves, gain control over the breath, and align the body. It also develops an appreciation for your body, your sole and singular vocal instrument. Always listen to your body.

Body awareness and a keener kinesthetic sense are more beneficial byproducts of yoga. Bring yoga to life in your life and you will reap its many rewards. And as long as you keep practicing, the rewards will remain. Yoga is not a solution or an ending point. Like learning to sing or making music, it is a continually evolving process, an exciting and ongoing journey, an abiding path that endures as it leads us, in the words of Iyengar, to "health, a sense of physical lightness, steadiness, clearness of countenance and a beautiful voice."[23]

Namaste!

Breathe,
Sing,
Be Free.

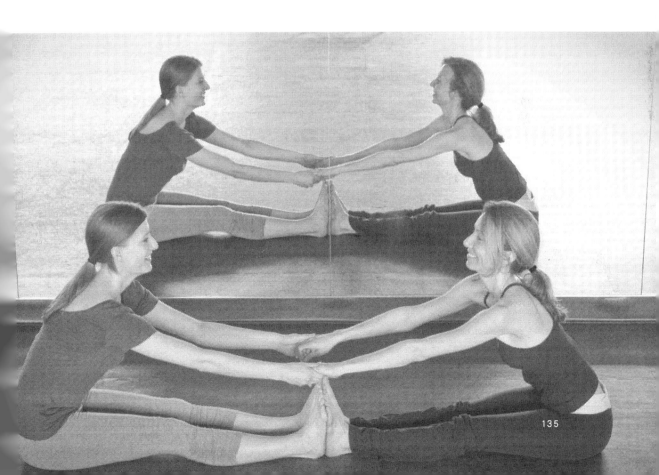

# Yoga Prescriptions for Singers

| Issue | Yoga Prescription |
|---|---|
| Tongue tension | Lion pose, Shitali breath |
| Jaw tension | Matangi mudra, Lion pose |
| Dry mouth | Bhudi mudra |
| Congestion/sinusitis | Shoulder stand/Plow pose, Breath of Fire, Bellows Breath |
| Low energy | Breath of Fire, Bellows breath, Chair pose, Warrior 2, Prana mudra |
| Nervous, rapid breathing | Shitali breath, Ujjayi breath |
| Weak, shallow inhalation | Kala breath, Uttarabodhi mudra |
| Lack of focus | Tree pose, L pose, Shoulder stand/Plow pose, Alternate nostril breathing, Jnana mudra, Toning or humming |
| Collapsed sternum | Reverse plank pose, Camel pose, Warrior 1 and Reverse Warrior pose, Cow face pose, Fish pose |
| Collapsed rib cage | Gate pose, Side Angle and Reverse Side Angle pose, Triangle and Revolved Triangle pose, Warrior 2 pose |
| Rounded spine | Cow pose, Cobra pose, Locust pose, Bow pose, Up Dog pose, Forward bends |

| Issue | Yoga Prescription |
|---|---|
| Poor alignment | Mountain pose, Plank pose, Warrior 3 pose, Bridge pose |
| Shoulder tension | Child pose, Down Dog pose, Cow face pose, Cat pose |
| Tight hips | Bound angle pose, Half or Full Lotus pose |

# EAT, DRINK, SING, AND DO YOGA

Just like practicing singing on a full stomach is not comfortable, practicing yoga after eating a big meal is not recommended. Asanas such as Locust, Cobra, and Bow are done lying on one's stomach, thus they cannot be completed comfortably while the digestive organs are busy processing food. (Not surprisingly, these belly poses are not meant for pregnant women and should not be part of any pre-natal yoga practice.)

Proper hydration is vital to both singing and yoga. Bikram or "sweaty" yoga causes profound perspiration and practitioners should be vigilant about preventing excessive fluid loss leading to dehydration. In any style of yoga, it is important to listen to your body and drink water before, during, and/or after yoga practice as feels best. I love a cup of chai tea before morning yoga practice. In fact, many modern yoga studios include tea rooms serving organic, herbal, and green tea.

# References

Bachman, Nicolai. *The Language of Yoga: Complete A to Y Guide to Asana Names, Sanskrit Terms, and Chants.* Louisville, CO: Sounds True, 2005.

Blades-Zeller, Elizabeth. *A Spectrum of Voices: Prominent American Voice Teachers Discuss the Teaching of Singing.* Lanham, MD: Scarecrow Press, 2003.

Brown, Jason Robert. *The Last Five Years.* New York: Hal Leonard, 2003.

Clark, Mark Ross. *Singing, Acting, and Movement in Opera: A Guide to Singer-getics.* Bloomington: Indiana University Press, 2002.

Emmons, Shirlee and Alma Thomas. *Power Performance for Singers: Transcending the Barriers.* New York: Oxford University Press, 1998.

Gass, Robert with Kathleen Brehony. *Chanting: Discovering Spirit in Sound.* New York: Broadway Books, 1999.

Gawain, Shakti. *Creative Visualization: Use the Power of Your Imagination to Create What You Want in Your Life.* Novato, CA: Nataraj Publishing, 2002.

Green, Barry with W. Timothy Gallwey. *The Inner Game of Music.* New York: Doubleday Books, 1986.

Harrison, George. *Chant and Be Happy! Indian Devotional Songs.* London: Apple Records, 1991.

Hines, Jerome. *Great Singers on Great Singing: A Famous Opera Star Interviews 40 Famous Opera Singers on the Technique of Singing.* New York: Limelight, 1984.

Hirschi, Gertrud. *Mudras: Yoga in Your Hands.* Boston: Weiser Books, 2000.

Iyengar, B.K.S. *Light on Pranayama: The Yogic Art of Breathing.* New York: Crossroad Publishing, 2004.

Iyengar, B.K.S. *Light on Yoga.* New York: Schocken Books, 1979.

Khalsa, Guru Dharam S. and Darryl O'Keeffe. *The Kundalini Yoga Experience: Bringing Body, Mind, and Spirit Together.* New York: Fireside, 2002.

Lee, Cyndi. *Yoga Body, Buddha Mind.* New York: Riverhead Books, 2004.

McKinney, James C. *The Diagnosis and Correction of Vocal Faults: A Manual for Teachers of Singing and for Choir Directors.* Long Grove, IL: Waveland Press, 2005.

Paul, Russill. *The Yoga of Sound: Tapping the Hidden Power of Music and Chant.* Novato, CA: New World Library, 2004.

Piper, Watty. *The Little Engine that Could.* New York: Platt and Munk, 1930.

Walden, Patricia. *Yoga Journal's Yoga Practice for Flexibility.* Broomfield, CO: Healing Arts, 1992.

# STICKING WITH YOGA

Committing to a yoga class is the best way to make yoga part of your training as a singer. But not everyone has access to (or money for) an organized class. Some may prefer to practice at home. If you don't want to buy yoga DVDs, you can rent them from Blockbuster or Netflix, or borrow them from the public library. Or try doing some yoga with Wii Fit! Or download Yoga Journal's iPractice iPhone application so you can instantly access fifteen different vinyasas.

Working with a partner can be fun and can help make you accountable for your yoga practice. Like having a jogging buddy or personal trainer, doing asanas with a partner is bonding (safety in numbers) and entertaining (remember playing Twister?). Furthermore, a partner can help you stretch deeper into the poses.

To help stay motivated, track your progress in a journal ("Today I finally touched my toes in seated forward bend. Bye-bye yoga strap!") or your facebook status! ("Megs has mastered her Warrior Three.")

# Ideas For Further Reading

Caponigro, Andy. *The Miracle of the Breath: Mastering Fear, Healing Illness, and Experiencing the Divine*. Novato, CA: New World Library, 2005.

Cheng, Stephen Chun-Tao. *The Tao of Voice: A New East-West Approach to Transforming the Singing and Speaking Voice*. Rochester, VT: Destiny Books, 1991.

Chopra, Deepak and Adam Plack. *The Soul of Healing Meditations*. New York: Rasa Music, 2001.

Chopra, Deepak and David Simon. *The Seven Spiritual Laws of Yoga*. Hoboken, NJ: John Wiley and Sons, 2004.

Cope, Stephen. *Yoga and the Quest for the True Self*. New York: Bantam Books, 1999.

Gilbert, Elizabeth. *Eat, Pray, Love: One Woman's Search for Everything Across Italy, India, and Indonesia*. New York: Penguin Books, 2006.

Levin-Gervasi, Stephanie. *The Smart Guide to Yoga*. New York: John Wiley and Sons, 1999.

McCall, Timothy. *Yoga as Medicine: The Yoga Prescription for Health and Healing*. New York: Bantam Books, 2007.

Melton, Joan with Kenneth Tom. *One Voice: Integrating Singing Technique and Theatre Voice Training*. Portsmouth, NH: Heinemann, 2003.

Pargman, David. *Managing Performance Stress: Models and Methods*. New York: Routledge, 2006.

Ristad, Eloise. *A Soprano on Her Head: Right-Side-Up Reflections on Life and Other Performances*. Boulder: CO: Real People Press, 1981.

# YOGA ISN'T JUST FOR GIRLS: REAL MEN EAT QUICHE AND DO YOGA

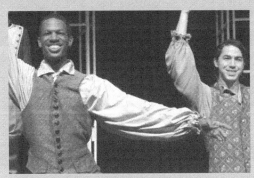

Jahi Mims (left) and Anthony Chu (right), in *The Merry Widow*

The benefits of yoga in forging a more healthy body and mind are well-established, and the deeper benefit of yoga in harnessing one's vocal instrument is the goal of this book. One of the best things about yoga is its universal application to both men and women. Yet even to this day there is still the notion that makes participation by men a sometimes nerve-wracking experience for them. Although ancient yoga gurus always seem to have been male, the modern prevalence of female practitioners has fed the idea that yoga is emasculating. Though very real in some would-be practitioners' minds, this notion couldn't be further from the truth. And thankfully time and culture are diminishing this issue.

Two students in my Yoga For Singers class, Anthony Chu and Jahi Mims, shared some insights into their immersion into yoga as men. "Taking yoga was a small emotional hurdle," replied Jahi. "I began taking it in high school, in a dance class that integrated yoga and Pilates. I was fully aware of the stigma that yoga was 'solely for women,' and since the class was mainly female, I did feel that stigma was reinforced." That would change, however, once Jahi would attend college with a bit more enlightened group of students assembled to experience a broad, liberal arts education. "The reactions from my male friends in college have been kind and respectful, and the women I've encountered have not been close-minded about my participation. I no longer have to flinch when I do yoga!"

Anthony's experience with the Yoga For Singers class corroborates Jahi's collegiate experience. "When speaking to my female friends there is really no talk about how strange it is for me to be doing yoga," said Anthony. "They actually are very supportive and encouraging. Also, when speaking with male friends, there really is no tension in our conversations about yoga. I even spoke with a baseball player who was interested in taking the yoga class." Indeed, yoga is becoming a more popular pursuit for students involved in college and high school athletics, with ever-increasing numbers of coaches and trainers encouraging their athletes to involve themselves in yoga under professional supervision. This breakthrough has led to a broader acceptance of yoga as practiced by men.

# Internet Resources

ABC-of-Yoga. A handy site, especially for its animated asana demonstrations. Free site membership entitles you to set up a personal profile and participate in forums and discussions and picture-sharing à la Facebook. http://www.abc-of-yoga.com/

CorePower Yoga. www.corepoweryoga.com Online yoga classes available 24 hours a day streaming online through subscription to Yoga On Demand. Podcasts are also available.

Elsie's online Yoga classes. www.elsiesyogakula.com Free online yoga classes also available for podcast. Teacher Elsie, a former actress, brings an Anusara emphasis to her practice. This is a great place to start if yoga classes or DVDs aren't in your budget or if you're a beginner intimidated by a group setting.

Spirit Sound. www.spiritsound.com Opera singer/voice teacher David Gordon has created an interesting website with a number of articles about Nada yoga and its benefits.

Svatmarama, Swami. *Hatha Yoga Pradipika.* A free online English translation of the classic text is available at: http://www.yogavidya.com/Yoga/HathaYogaPradipika.pdf

Yoga.com www.yoga.com This is a good all-purpose yoga site with a helpful studio/teacher directory (by zip code). Other nice parts of the site include the yoga pose of the month and attractive yoga desktop backgrounds and screensavers.

Yoga Journal. www.yogajournal.com Yoga Journal is a wonderful magazine and their website is a great resource. It provides a useful glossary of poses. Asanas are clearly described and best of all, their benefits and contraindications are listed as well as recommended variations, modifications, preparatory and follow-up poses. The site also features the hilarious Inappropriate Yoga Guy, Ogden.

YOGAmazing.com With a focus on vinyasa yoga, founder Chaz Rough provides weekly free podcasts on iTunes. He often relates how yoga is helpful to various sports, but he is also a singer/song-writer.

Yogasite.com www.yogasite.com This is a well-rounded online reference site and resource center with articles, merchandise, and a calendar of workshops on an international level.

Yogadownload.com. A wide mix of classes from the basics to more obscure Jivamukti and Forrest Yoga as well as Yoga for Cyclists, Runners, Back Pain, Kids, and Yoga with Weights. You can also customize your own class.

Other sites for online yoga classes:
myyogaonline.com, yogaclass.com, yogalearningcenter.com, yogatoday.com

---

*"I was skeptical, to say the least. I was wary of the clichés associated with yoga: spirituality used as a marketing tool or Eastern philosophy sold at Starbucks to disenchanted lawyers and accountants looking for meaning. What I soon realized is that yoga welcomes everyone. Yoga will drastically improve you in every way imaginable."*

—**Adam Levine**, *lead singer of Maroon 5*

# Sample Yoga Playlist:
## For Class Use or Solo Practice

| | | |
|---|---|---|
| **Frou Frou** | *Let Go* | A liberating class opener for initial asanas and starting stretches. |
| **U2** | *Breathe* | A powerful, energizing song for Sun Salutations. |
| **Michelle Branch** | *Breathe* | Another vitalizing selection which helps promote prana. |
| **Jason Mraz** | *The Remedy* | The remedy is avoiding apprehension in life, and in challenging poses like Revolved Triangle. |
| **Alanis Morissette** | *Incomplete* | An important reminder to focus on the process and progress of your practice, and your life. |
| **Mat Kearney** | *Breathe In, Breathe Out* | This song helps equalize inhalation and exhalation as in Kala breathing. |
| **Idina Menzel** | *Defying Gravity* | An apt accompaniment to balancing poses such as Tree, Eagle, and Warrior III. |
| **U2** | *Walk On* | Bono reassures you to leave behind heartache and open your heart into forward bends. |
| **Ingrid Michaelsen** | *Keep Breathing* | Remember not to hold your breath as you begin to arch the back into Bridge and Wheel. |
| **The Beatles** | *Let It Be* | This zen-like mantra clears the mind in Shoulder Stand and Plow. |
| **Taylor Swift** | *Breathe* | Release negative energy through long exhalations and deep spinal twists. |
| **Sarah McLachlan** | *Perfect Girl* | Perfect for closing Corpse pose meditation with its soothing paean on patience and self-acceptance. |

# Jazz Yoga Playlist:

## For those who want a little swing to their practice

| | | |
|---|---|---|
| **Nikki Yanofsky** | *On the Sunny Side of the Street* | For your starting Sun Salutations. |
| **Diana Krall** | *Pick Yourself Up* | Pick yourself up from Up Dog to Down Dog. |
| **Michael Bublé** | *Feeling Good* | Your shoulders will feel good after Cat pose and Thread the Needle. |
| **Natalie Cole** | *Straighten Up and Fly Right* | Straighten your spine as you fly into Eagle or Crow pose. |
| **Esperanza Spalding** | *Fall In* | Don't be afraid of falling as you balance in Warrior Three. |
| **Norah Jones** | *Light as a Feather* | A spiritual song about the oneness of the world. |
| **Jamie Cullum** | *What a Difference a Day Makes* | Doing daily yoga can make a difference in your vocal health and emotional well-being. |
| **Jane Monheit** | *Lucky to Be Me* | Gratitude is a vital yogic concept. |
| **Tierney Sutton** | *The Best is Yet to Come* | Look forward to your next pose and your next performance. |
| **Peter Cincotti** | *Lay Your Body Down (Goodbye Philadelphia)* | Lay yourself down for Locust or Bow pose. |
| **Harry Connick Jr.** | *Let Me Love Tonight* | Roll onto your back and use this soothing song for spinal twists. |
| **Dianne Reeves** | *Olokun* | Mystical music for mantra meditation. |

# PLAYLIST POSSIBILITIES

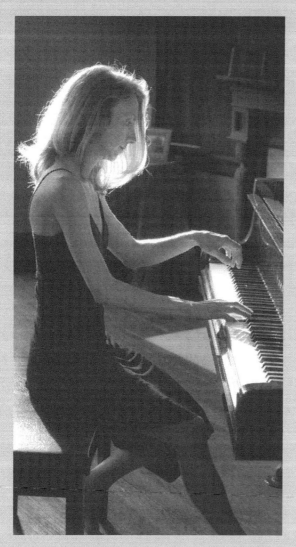

Devising your own yoga playlists can be a fun way to enhance and personalize your practice. Select a theme or pick your preferred genre, then compile and collate your favorite tunes. Perhaps you are inspired by Gospel Yoga (i.e. Jennifer Hudson's powerful voice) or Bluegrass Yoga (ethereal Allison Krauss); or maybe Emo Yoga provides catharsis or you find transcendence via Movie Soundtrack Yoga (haunting *American Beauty* or hypnotic *Inception*).

Voice major Ali Wreggelsworth thinks that "doing yoga to Disney music would be amazing!" Indeed a mix of Disney Princess anthems could be empowering, and the *Tinker Bell* album contains a wealth of uplifting songs (like "Let Your Heart Sing").

Although he also appreciates Disney, Knoxville Opera vocal coach/répétiteur Patrick Harvey has operatic ideas for his ideal yoga playlist: the exquisite *Rosenkavalier* Trio by Richard Strauss and Humperdinck's heavenly dream ballet from *Hansel and Gretel*. You could even meditate to Massenet's Meditation from *Thaïs*.

# Adam Levine's Yoga Playlist
## (featured in Women's Health)

| | |
|---|---|
| **Quinton Tarver and Lee Perry** | *Time After Time* |
| **Al Green** | *Tired Of Being Alone* |
| **D'Angelo** | *Brown Sugar* |
| **Jill Scott** | *A Long Walk* |
| **Marvin Gaye** | *What's Goin' On* |
| **Lupe Fiasco** | *Kick Push* |
| **Amy Winehouse** | *You Know That I'm No Good* |
| **Jem** | *Maybe I'm Amazed* |
| **Natalie Merchant** | *Life is Sweet* |
| **Norah Jones** | *Turn Me On* |
| **Peter Gabriel** | *Games Without Frontiers* |
| **Seal** | *Love's Divine* |
| **Maxwell** | *Whenever, Wherever, Whatever* |
| **Sweet** | *We Are One* |

*"Yoga for Singers vastly improved my singing technique. It helped to correct my habit of singing in a slumped-over posture, in turn alleviating some of the breathing issues I dealt with. Yoga for Singers also taught me ways to relax. For someone who gets extremely nervous and tense before performing, learning to relax myself in a few simple moves was a huge breakthrough. I highly recommend yoga for any singer regardless of their technical level, because it promotes the healthy lifestyle that is so important to us."*

—**Hope Moore**, *BM in music education*

# WHAT DID YFS DO FOR YOU?

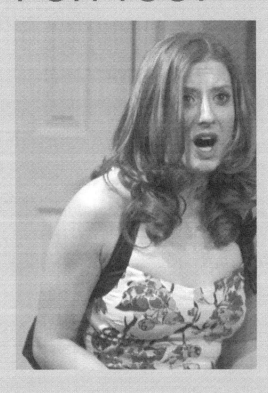

Before taking the Yoga For Singers class, I had dabbled in yoga, but it wasn't a regular practice for me. I had been interested enough to learn some poses, but didn't get any farther than that. It wasn't until I took the class that I realized what it could offer me as a singer. The good habits that I developed in the class have stayed with me – and not just for my voice training but also for maintaining my physical well-being.

The first place I saw results with my yoga regimen was in auditioning. When singing, there are certain occasions – such as auditions and jury performances– that have always gotten the best of me. Step in front of an audience, trying to prove myself as a singer, and I become a nervous wreck! But through breathing exercises and the use of specific poses, YFS taught me to calm my nerves and approach performing with serenity, becoming an integral part of my auditioning ritual.

Also through YFS, I learned poses – like the Warriors, forward bends and spinal twists – that helped me realign my posture before singing. After doing these types of poses, it's almost like pressing "reset" on my posture – when I come back up, I'm all set physically. It's kind of like wiping the slate clean of any physical tension, as my body is now reminded of where it needs to be. Needless to say, this opens up my vocal instrument so I can sing better.

I took YFS for two years, and the skills, poses, and vinyasas I learned have made me a much calmer person. I know I can always go to it if I am feeling lethargic and in need of reenergizing myself. Without it, I'd almost certainly be falling into bad physical habits, as my body would default into the kinds of positions that would keep me from reaching my fullest potential. I am able to use the tools I learned in Yoga For Singers in the very moments I need it most, and it has made me a better, more confident singer.

–Megs Free, BFA in Musical Theatre

# Glossary: Sanskrit Terms

## Pronunciation guide in International Phonetic Alphabet (IPA)

| | | |
|---|---|---|
| *Asana* | ['asana] | Literally, seat. A yoga pose or position. |
| *Chakra* | ['ʧakra] | Literally, wheel or circle. Energy meridian or wheel in the body. |
| *Dharana* | ['dara'na] | Focus, concentration. |
| *Dhyana* | ['ʤana] | Meditation. |
| *Ekagrata* | [E'kagrata] | Fixing on one point. |
| *Hatha* | ['hata] | Literally, sun and moon. Physical yoga. Americanized to [haΘa] |
| *Kapalabhati* | [ka'palabati] | Breath of Fire. |
| *Kumbhaka* | ['kumbaka] | Retention of air after inhalation and before exhalation. |
| *Kundalini* | ['kunda'lini] | Literally, coiled. Psychic energy coiled in the spine like a snake. |
| *Mantra* | ['mantra] | Literally, mind deliverance. A repeated word/phrase of affirmation. |
| *Mudra* | [mu'dra] | Literally, seal. A symbolic hand gesture used in meditation. |
| *Namaste* | [namas'de] | Literally, I bow to you. A traditional yoga greeting or thank you. |

| | | |
|---|---|---|
| *Prana* | ['prana] | Life, breath, or energy. |
| *Pranayama* | [prana'jama] | Literally, life control. Breath control techniques. |
| *Pratyahara* | [pratja'hara] | Withdrawal of the senses. |
| *Puraka* | ['puraka] | Inhalation. |
| *Rechaka* | ['rEʧaka] | Exhalation. |
| *Samadhi* | [sa'madhi] | State of perfection; higher level of meditation. |
| *Shamatha* | [ʃa'mata] | Literally, peaceful abiding, as in meditation. |
| *Shitali* | ['ʃitali] | Cooling breath curling the sides of the tongue. |
| *Ujjayi* | [u'ʤai] | Victorious breath. |
| *Vinyasa* | [vin'jasa] | Literally, to place in a certain way. A sequence of asanas. |
| *Yoga* | ['joga] | Literally, yoking or joining. The union or communion of the body and mind. |

# Glossary: Styles/Schools of Yoga

| | | | |
|---|---|---|---|
| *Ananda yoga* | ['ananda] | Uses silent affirmations in asanas in this gentle, spiritual style. | www.anandayoga.org |
| *AntiGravity yoga* | | Combines yoga with acrobatics done in a soft trapeze known as an "AntiGravity hammock" with a focus on advanced inversions. | www.antigravityyoga.com |
| *Ashtanga yoga* | [aʃ'taŋga] | "Power yoga." Emphasizes intense vinyasas. | www.ashtanga.com |
| *Bikram yoga* | ['bIkram] | "Hot yoga." Done in a room heated to 105 degrees Farenheit with 40% humidity to sweat out toxins and assist flexibility. | www.bikramyoga.com |
| *Iyengar yoga* | [aI'jEngar] | Emphasizes alignment and using props to help form. | www.bksiyengar.com |
| *Kripalu yoga* | ['krIpaɭu] | Combines kundalini and pranayama with a focus on "body wisdom." | www.kripalu.org |
| *Kundalini yoga* | ['kunda'lini] | Vitalizes kundalini energy through asanas and chakra meditation. | www.kundaliniyoga.org |

| | | | |
|---|---|---|---|
| *Nada yoga* | [ 'nada ] | "Sound yoga," closely related to Shabda yoga. | |
| *Shabda yoga* | [ 'ʃabda ] | "Word yoga." Involves chanting of mantras and toning of vowels. | www.russillpaul.com |
| *Sivananda yoga* | [ ʃIva'nanda ] | Emphasizes lifestyle elements such as positive thinking and vegetarianism. | www.sivananda.org |
| *Viniyoga* | [ 'vInijoga ] | Focuses on function over form with a therapeutic emphasis. | www.viniyoga.com |
| *Yogilates* | [ jogI'latiz ] | Combines yoga with Pilates (based on toning the core abdominal muscles). | www.yogilates.com |
| *Yoga booty ballet* ® | | The latest yoga fusion fitness routine combining yoga and dance with toning focused on the abs and buttocks. | www.yogabootyballet.com |
| *YAS Yoga* | [ jæs ] | Yoga for Athletes. Geared towards improving sports performance and helping prevent injury. | www.go2yas.com |

# End Notes

[1] B.K.S. Iyengar, *Light on Yoga* (New York: Schocken Books, 1979): 22.

[2] Ibid, 40.

[3] Guru Dharam S. Khalsa and Darryl O'Keefe, *The Kundalini Yoga Experience: Bringing Body, Mind, and Spirit Together* (New York: Gaia Books, 2002): 11.

[4] James C. McKinney, *The Diagnosis and Correction of Vocal Faults: A Manual for Teachers of Singing and for Choir Directors* (Long Grove, IL: Waveland Press, 2005): 51.

[5] Iyengar, *Light on Pranayama: The Yogic Art of Breathing* (New York: Crossroad Publishing, 2004): 19.

[6] Ibid, 87.

[7] Ibid, 139.

[8] Ibid, 176, 265.

[9] Mark Ross Clark, *Singing, Dancing, and Movement in Opera: A Guide to Singer-getics* (Bloomington: Indiana University Press, 2002): 12.

[10] McKinney, 35, 55.

[11] Patricia Walden, *Yoga Journal's Yoga Practice for Flexibility* (Broomfield, CO: Healing Arts, 1992).

[12] Cyndi Lee, *Yoga Body, Buddha Mind* (New York: Riverhead Books, 2004): 13, 15.

[13] Ibid, 17-18.

[14] Shirlee Emmons and Alma Thomas, *Power Performance for Singers: Transcending the Barriers* (New York: Oxford University Press, 1998): 14.

[15] Iyengar, *Light on Yoga*, 48-49.

[16] Khalsa, 119.

[17] Shakti Gawain, *Creative Visualization* (Novato, CA: Nataraj Publishing, 2002): 31.

[18] Ibid, 31-33.

[19] Gertrud Hirschi, *Mudras: Yoga in your Hands* (Boston: Weiser Books, 2000): 26.

[20] Barry Green with W. Timothy Gallwey, *The Inner Game of Music*
(New York: Doubleday Books, 1986): 126-7.

[21] Robert Gass with Kathleen Brehony, *Chanting: Discovering Spirit in Sound*
(New York: Broadway Books, 1999): 45.

[22] Russill Paul, *The Yoga of Sound: Tapping the Hidden Power of Music and Chant*
(Novato, CA: New World Library, 2004): 78-79.

[23] Iyengar, *Light on Yoga*, 51.

# About The Author

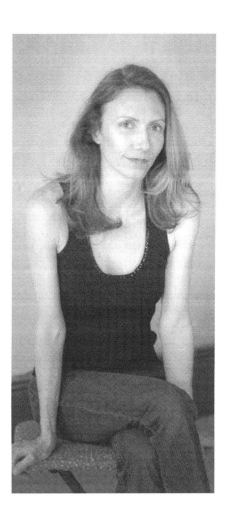

**LINDA LISTER** was educated at Vassar College, Cambridge University, and the Eastman School of Music. Her writings have been featured in the *Journal of Singing, Classical Singer Magazine, Voice Prints, Encyclopedia of American Music and Culture, American Music Teacher* and *Popular Music and Society* as well as the book *The Brontës in the World of the Arts* published by Ashgate in 2008. A certified CorePower Yoga teacher, she has presented workshops on Yoga for Singers throughout the country as well as at national conventions for the National Association of Teachers of Singing and the National Opera Association. Also a composer, she has written a number of vocal works including the chamber opera *How Clear She Shines!* Affectionately known as "Limber Lister," Linda is a voice professor and professional singer in the genres of opera, musical theatre, jazz, lieder, and mélodie and is featured on the Albany Records CDs *The American Soloist* and *Midnight Tolls.* Of the roles she has performed onstage, some of her favorites include Musetta in *La Bohème,* Adina in *The Elixir of Love,* Massenet's *Cinderella,* Maggie in *A Chorus Line,* and Woman 1 in *Songs for a New World,* as well as Madge in the world premiere of Libby Larsen's opera *Picnic.* In 2011, Linda became the Director of UNLV Opera Theatre.

www.lindalister.com
yogaforsingers@gmail.com

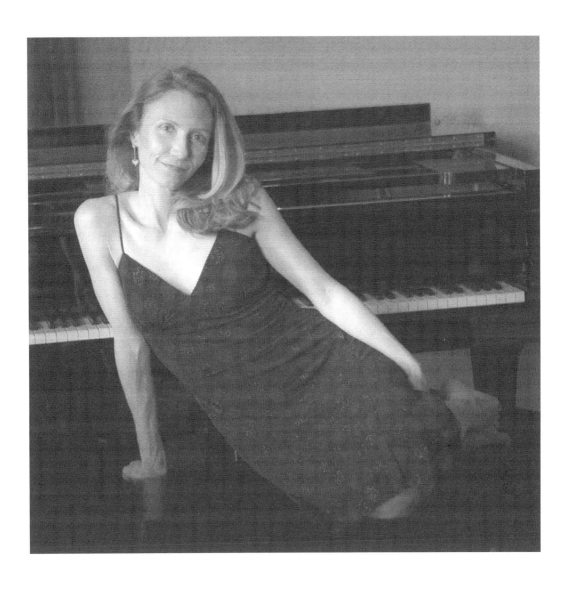

*"The Song is You."*

— *Oscar Hammerstein II*